Top Screwups
Doctors Make and
How to Avoid Them

Top Screwups Doctors Make and How to Avoid Them

Joe Graedon, MS, and Teresa Graedon, PhD

CROWN ARCHETYPE

NEW YORK

Library of Congress Cataloging-in-Publication Data

Graedon, Joe.
Top screwups doctors make and how to avoid them /
Joe Graedon & Teresa Graedon.—1st ed.
        p.   cm.
1. Medical errors.   I. Graedon, Teresa, 1947–   II. Title.
R729.8.G73 2011
610.28'9—dc23   2011016332

ISBN 978-0-307-46091-2
eISBN 978-0-307-46093-6

PRINTED IN THE UNITED STATES OF AMERICA

Jacket design by Nupoor Gordon

3   5   7   9   10   8   6   4   2

This Book Is Dedicated to
the Memory of Helen Graedon

Who lived her life with courage, compassion, enthusiasm,
and perseverance. Her love and support nourished us over the decades.
We hope this book will mean that her tragic death was not in vain.

and

To health care providers who strive to offer patients safe, effective,
and compassionate care.

Contents

Acknowledgments

The patient safety movement has taken root. There are now many physicians, nurses, pharmacists, and other health care providers working diligently to improve the current disastrous situation. There is a great deal of work to be done, but these pioneering souls are leading the way through their research, outreach, and direct interaction with patients.

It isn't possible to list all the people who have in some way contributed to our understanding of the scope of the problem and the steps needed for improvement. Here are just some of the individuals who have helped make this book possible directly or indirectly. We also want to acknowledge all the patients and family members who have contributed their stories through our newspaper column, radio show, and website.

Jerry Avorn, MD, is one of the country's leading experts in drug safety. His innovative research has helped us understand some of the pitfalls in clinical trials. We are especially grateful for his attention to the problems that drugs can pose for older people.

David Bates, MD, is one of the pioneers in the patient safety movement. We are grateful for his research and his efforts to move his colleagues forward.

Steven Feldman, MD, PhD, is a dermatologist who has thought long and hard about the issues of communication between physicians and patients and the ways it can go awry. We recommend his book *Compartments: How the Brightest, Best Trained, and Most Caring People Can Make Judgments That Are Completely and Utterly Wrong.*

Karen Frush, MD, is chief patient safety officer for the Duke University Health System and is one of many Duke physicians working hard to make the institution a safer place. We are grateful for her efforts.

Curt Furberg, MD, PhD, is an outspoken advocate for drug safety. His integrity and dedication make him one of our heroes.

Nortin Hadler, MD, is one of the smartest analysts of medical practice that we know. He opened our eyes to the many ways statistics can be used to mislead physicians and patients alike. We highly recommend his book *Worried Sick: A Prescription for Health in an Overtreated America.*

Heather Jackson is an editor who has led us hither and yon and who immediately understood the importance of this book. We are extremely grateful for the opportunity that she created.

Sydny Miner is a marvelous editor who picked up where Heather Jackson left off and helped us to move this project forward with great insight and skill.

Thomas Moore is senior research scientist at the Institute for Safe Medication Practices. His success at cracking the code for the Food and Drug Administration's Adverse Event Reporting System and his passion for discussing drug safety have contributed greatly to our thinking.

Robert Muder, MD, is a professor of medicine at the University of Pittsburgh in the Division of Infectious Diseases and the chief of the Infectious Disease Section at the Veterans Affairs Pittsburgh Healthcare System. He helped us understand how patients can be protected from health care–acquired infections.

David Newman-Toker, MD, PhD, is a neurologist and colleague with Peter Pronovost at the Johns Hopkins University School of Medicine.

His landmark paper (with Peter Pronovost) in the *Journal of the American Medical Association* ("Diagnostic Errors—The Next Frontier for Patient Safety") opened our eyes to one of the top screwups in medicine today. Dr. Newman-Toker's groundbreaking research in developing a fast, inexpensive strategy for diagnosing strokes (*Stroke,* November 2009) is the kind of innovative thinking we admire.

Art Papier, MD, is an innovative dermatologist who, with his colleague Lowell Goldsmith, MD, came up with a brilliant way to help health care providers and patients diagnose skin problems. Dr. Papier provided the spark that lit the fire that illuminated this book.

Peter Pronovost, MD, PhD, is our hero. He has made patient safety a cornerstone of his career and is renowned for his innovative work developing the "checklist" concept for medicine. Dr. Pronovost speaks truth to power. He is a professor at the Johns Hopkins University School of Medicine, where he directs the Quality and Safety Research Group and serves as the medical director of the Center for Innovation in Quality Care. We highly recommend his book *Safe Patients, Smart Hospitals: How One Doctor's Checklist Can Help Change Health Care from the Inside Out.*

Lisa Sanders, MD, is a fantastic physician-communicator. Her articles on diagnosis for the *New York Times Magazine* alerted us to the human side of diagnostic error. We highly recommend her book *Every Patient Tells a Story: Medical Mysteries and the Art of Diagnosis.*

Charlotte Sheedy is first and foremost an exceptional human being. She is also an amazing book agent who initially saw the value of this work even more clearly than we did. Her support and encouragement over the last decades has been crucial to our writing.

Robert Wachter, MD, is another giant in the field of patient safety. His insights have been extremely helpful to us in this project, and we highly recommend his book *Internal Bleeding: The Truth Behind America's Terrifying Epidemic of Medical Mistakes.*

Larry Weed, MD, is a legend and an innovative thinker who was thirty years ahead of his colleagues. He is still way out in front of most of his colleagues when it comes to thinking creatively about medical education, diagnosis, and treatment.

Raymond Woosley, MD, PhD, is a drug safety expert who has been at the forefront of investigating drug interactions for decades.

Top Screwups
Doctors Make and
How to Avoid Them

PREFACE

The panicked phone call from my mother awakened me from a dead sleep at 2:00 A.M. "Joe, I've been poisoned! Come quick, I'm in terrible trouble." I had left her side at Duke Hospital in Durham, North Carolina, only a few hours earlier after she had undergone a successful angioplasty of one coronary artery.

Although Helen Graedon was ninety-two years old, ate meat and potatoes her entire life, and did not believe in vigorous exercise, the arteries in her heart were in amazingly good condition, all except for one. The interventional cardiologist at Duke had opened that one with ease and was delighted with the outcome. When I left her room around 9:00 P.M. that evening, she was feeling fine and looking forward to coming home the next morning.

When I arrived at her bedside a little after 2:00 A.M., she was indeed in terrible trouble. She was agitated and scared. The nurses had tied her legs to the bed. Even so, she was thrashing around wildly, her muscles in constant spasm. She told me again that she had been poisoned. When I asked the nurse what had happened, she said that at 10:00 P.M., my mother had been given the narcotic pain reliever Demerol (meperidine) and the sedating antihistamine Phenergan (promethazine) but insisted that her extreme distress could not have been caused by the medicines.

I knew my mother could not tolerate narcotics. Only five hours earlier, I had made a point of telling the same nurse and the intern on duty that my mother must never be given morphine or any other narcotic. That information was in her medical chart, too. The trouble was, they didn't have her chart handy, and no one bothered to tell the resident who came by at 10:00 P.M. to remove the sheath from her femoral artery not to administer a narcotic. Instead, he injected Demerol because it was the standard protocol after such procedures. It likely interacted with another medication she had been taking and led to agitation, uncontrollable muscle contractions, and, ultimately, her death.

I spent the next four hours holding her hand, comforting her, and watching helplessly as her body was wracked by convulsive movements and shrieks of terror. Gradually, as the drug effects began to wear off, she started to relax, and eventually she was able to doze off and get a little sleep. I knew something very bad had happened, but I was too exhausted to think clearly.

By morning, she seemed somewhat recovered, and the attending physician told me I would be able to take her home around noon. Just as I was getting ready to come pick her up, a call came from the hospital. Helen had fallen on the way to the bathroom, I was told, and was near death. I sped to the hospital, only to arrive a few minutes after she had died.

My mother had recently developed drug-induced diabetes and heart failure. She knew her days were numbered. But she should not have died in such a tragic way on December 14, 1996. She should have been going home to recuperate from a successful angioplasty procedure.

Instead, a series of medical errors led to the horrific conclusion of a wonderful life. The anticoagulant she was given during her angioplasty was contraindicated for someone who had recently suffered a serious bleeding episode—she had hemorrhaged less than ten days earlier when she was given an experimental drug during a prior hospital stay. In addition, the Demerol interacted with a medicine she was taking, Eldepryl (selegiline for mood), to produce "serotonin syndrome"; this condition is marked by uncontrollable muscle contractions, restlessness, and agitation.

The death certificate stated that Helen Graedon's death was caused by "cardiac arrest" due to "hypotension" (low blood pressure) as a consequence of "retroperitoneal hemorrhage" (internal bleeding). What it did *not* say was that the uncontrollable muscle contractions the night before almost certainly brought on the hemorrhaging. Duke physicians later told us that bleeding at the site in the groin where the catheter is passed into the femoral artery is a major concern after angioplasty. The most important way to reduce this problem, we were told by the Duke cardiologists: *"The patient must lie still."*

We could have sued Duke Hospital for the series of mistakes that were made that led to my mother's death. In addition to administering inappropriate medications, they also placed her walker out of reach but left the side rail on her bed down and did not have a nurse available to help her to the bathroom. When a proud woman tried to make it without assistance, she fell. With such low blood pressure from internal bleeding, she died within minutes. No one volunteered information on the events leading to her demise other than to tell us that she had fallen. We pieced together the rest of the story on our own.

A high-powered malpractice attorney said we had a clear case of negligence and harm. He also told us that Duke was unlikely to change its practices even if we were to win. So instead of a lawsuit, we began a long campaign to try to reduce medical errors and improve patient safety at Duke Hospital. For more than a decade, we have been working to change the system and make it safer. We have served on the Duke Patient Safety and Clinical Quality Committee of the Board of Trustees and also on the Patient Advocacy Council. Our goal has been to reduce medical errors and make Duke a more patient-centered institution. It has been a slow and frustrating process. Institutions are slow to change, but we have worked with dedicated doctors and staff to make this health system better. Duke is in many ways a much safer place than it was on the night of December 13, 1996. We wish we could say with confidence that such a tragedy could never happen again. We can't.

U.S. News and World Report considered nearly five thousand medical centers in the United States in 2010–11. Duke University Medical Center ranked number ten on the Honor Role of Best Hospitals, ahead of the prestigious Brigham and Women's Hospital in Boston. Duke Hospital is clearly one of the country's finest medical institutions. Nevertheless, lethal errors have been made.

Since my mother's death, a young Mexican American woman, Jesica Santillan, received a mismatched heart during a transplant operation at Duke and died. A baby was accidentally burned in the neonatal intensive care unit. Thousands of surgical patients were exposed to used elevator fluid during surgery because the fluid was mistakenly put in old detergent containers. The instruments were then washed with this hydraulic fluid instead of detergent. Those are just the Duke cases that have achieved media attention.

Duke does not stand alone. Serious mistakes are made at every hospital in America on a daily basis. Although we have spent more than thirty-five years trying to prevent drug interactions and complications for others, we could not save a woman we loved. We cannot share what we have learned about safety and quality efforts at the Duke University Health System. We signed a confidentiality agreement and cannot relate what goes on behind closed doors. We can tell you that many hospitals bury their mistakes, metaphorically and sometimes literally. Out of fear of lawsuits, hospitals resist public disclosure of medical mistakes. This keeps other health care providers from learning about errors and preventing the same exact problems from happening at their institutions.

Highlighting the most common, preventable errors in hospitals, doctors' offices and pharmacies will, we hope, give you the information and tools you need to help prevent these errors and protect yourself and those you love. This book distills the lessons we have learned over three decades so that you can benefit from them.

SAFE PATIENT CHECKLIST

Our goal in writing this book is to help you avoid a medical mistake for yourself or someone you love. As you will learn, errors are common and often preventable. As many as one in three patients will experience an error during a hospital stay.[1] We do *not* want to discourage you from seeking appropriate health care, but we *do* want to offer you tools to make such encounters as safe as possible.

Assume that mistakes will be made, whether you are seeing your primary care provider, consulting a specialist, or being treated in the hospital. Your mission is to detect potential errors before they can do you damage.

In almost every chapter you will discover a "top 10" list of screwups to avoid or tips to protect yourself. Here is our overview of some key strategies for safer health care:

✓ Take a prioritized list of your top health concerns/symptoms.

✓ Ask the doctor for a recap to make sure you have been heard.

✓ Take notes or record the conversation: you won't remember everything you have heard.

✓ Take a friend or family member to be your advocate and record keeper.

✓ Get a list of all your medications and supplements so that interactions can be prevented.

✓ Find out about the most common and serious side effects your medications may cause.

✓ Ask the doctor how confident he or she is about your diagnosis. Find out what else could cause your symptoms.

✓ When in doubt, seek a second opinion.

✓ Always ask your providers to wash their hands before they examine you.

✓ Get your medical records and test results.

✓ Keep track of your progress: maintain a diary of relevant measurements such as weight, blood pressure, and blood sugar readings.

✓ Be especially vigilant when moving from one health care setting to another. Mistakes and oversights are especially common during transitions.

✓ Ask how to get in touch with your providers. Get phone numbers or e-mail addresses, and learn when to report problems.

✓ Inquire about resources to learn more about your diagnosis or treatment.

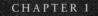

CHAPTER 1

INTRODUCTION

Statistics are people with the tears wiped away. —IRVING SELIKOFF, MD

Imagine the headlines today if a jumbo jet crashed and killed everyone on board. Now imagine three jumbo jets crashing on the same day. There would be cries of outrage, demands for explanations, investigations, and immediate corrections to air traffic safety.

The death toll from health care screwups adds up to at least 500,000 Americans annually. That is the equivalent of more than three jumbo jets crashing *every day of the year* (or over 1,000 jets annually). Because these individuals are dying at home, in hospitals, or in nursing homes, no one is counting the bodies. There is no outrage, no plan to change a system that allows too many to die unnecessarily. The medical profession seems largely immune to the consequences of its errors.

If our calculations are correct, it means that medical mistakes are the third leading cause of death in the United States, right after heart disease (616,067) and cancer (562,875) and way ahead of strokes, the next big killer (135,952).[1] Teasing out the total number of people dying from health care errors turns out to be incredibly difficult. In the airline industry, when a plane crashes, the death toll is known almost immediately. But to figure out how many people die each year because of misdiagnosis, medication mistakes, preventable infections, oversights, suboptimal treatment, and just plain mess-ups, we need to consider a range of statistics. There is no one place to go for such data, and the estimates that we found vary enormously.

To Err Is Human

In 1999, an organization of the country's leading health experts issued an astonishing report titled *To Err Is Human*.[2] The Institute of Medicine (IOM), tasked with making unbiased policy recommendations to improve the health of Americans, estimated that as many as 98,000 citizens died each year in hospitals and 1 million patients were injured from a range of mistakes. The report created a firestorm of controversy inside and outside the medical community. There was a lot of hand wringing, a fair amount of denial, and eventually some brainstorming about how to improve things.

Five years later, two of the country's leading safety experts, Lucian Leape, MD, and Donald Berwick, MD, wrote a tough article in the *Journal of the American Medical Association* titled: "Five Years After *To Err Is Human*: What Have We Learned?" The answer: not much. Their conclusion: still no nationwide monitoring system and little evidence of patient safety improvement.[3]

Then came another bombshell. A leading independent health care ratings organization called HealthGrades reviewed Medicare data from hospitals around the country and concluded that the IOM report had grossly underestimated the number of deaths. The 2004 report concluded that the death rate was roughly twice the previous number, or an average of 195,000 citizens dying annually from preventable in-hospital medical errors.[4]

Another investigative report released by journalists from the Hearst Corporation in 2009, titled *Dead by Mistake*, estimated that 200,000 Americans died that year from hospital infections and preventable medical errors.[5] In 2010, an in-depth study from the Department of Health and Human Services estimated that 134,000 Medicare hospital patients are harmed from medical care each month and 180,000 die every year as a result.[6] Almost half the deaths were preventable. This mortality number includes only senior citizens, so the total annual mortality resulting from medical care is substantially higher.

More alarming than the incredible numbers of deaths was the

lobbying effort by the American Medical Association, the American Hospital Association, and other special-interest groups that blocked any organized system for reporting medical errors.[7] A decade after all the agonizing and brainstorming by eminent experts, we still lack a way of actually detecting and tracking medical screwups. According to Christopher Landrigan, MD, a leading patient safety investigator, "We need a monitoring system that is mandatory. There has to be some mechanism for federal-level reporting, where hospitals across the country are held to it."[8]

Without some sort of compulsory reporting system, hospitals may miss or ignore "93 percent of events that cause either permanent or temporary harm to a patient."[9] That was the conclusion the Inspector General of Health and Human Services made based on a careful review of 278 Medicare hospitalizations.[10] A 2010 study published in the *New England Journal of Medicine* revealed that harm to patients resulting from medical care remains common, even in places where significant resources have been devoted to improving safety.[11] Nearly one in five hospital patients in the study suffered harm, and two-fifths of those injuries could have been prevented.[12] A study in 2011 estimated that 6.1 million Americans are injured each year due to medical misadventures.[13]

Dead by Mistake Key Findings

- "20 states have no medical error reporting at all, five states have voluntary reporting systems and five are developing reporting systems.
- "Of the 20 states that require medical error reporting, hospitals report only a tiny percentage of their mistakes, standards vary wildly and enforcement is often nonexistent.
- "In terms of public disclosure, 45 states currently do not release hospital-specific information.
- "Only 17 states have systematic adverse-event reporting systems that are transparent enough to be useful to consumers."[14]

What these data mean is that we have no idea how many people are actually dying from medical mess-ups. And, dear reader, please note that everything we have been discussing until now has to do with hospitals. It does not include nursing homes (where oversight is far less rigorous and where mishaps rarely get reported) or outpatient settings such as urgent care centers, clinics, private offices, pharmacies, or surgical centers, where physicians and other health care providers have no requirement (and a disincentive) to acknowledge or report mistakes. Even in hospitals, doctors are far less likely to report medical errors than nurses. In one study, "registered nurses provided nearly half of the reports; physicians contributed less than 2 percent."[15] In another study of Massachusetts hospitals, physicians disclosed less than one-third of preventable adverse events.[16]

It would be reasonable to conclude that measuring medical mistakes is imprecise. In fact, research shows that "never events," that is, events that should never happen, are severely underreported. The Institute for Healthcare Improvement, an organization that promotes patient safety, has developed a standardized approach to reviewing patient records to detect signals of problems in medical care. This technique, known as the Global Trigger Tool, was used in one study to review approximately eight hundred patient records. The Global Trigger Tool identified more than 350 medical errors, while a computerized record review found thirty-five in the same set of records. Voluntary reporting had revealed only four of these mistakes. It's little wonder that the investigators concluded that relying on voluntary reporting alone could result in serious misjudgments of patient safety.[17] In fact, 33 percent of the patients in this study experienced adverse events. This is ten times more than prior studies have found.

The Tip of the Iceberg

As we did our research for this book, we began to sense we were seeing only the tip of the error iceberg. To get a more comprehensive overview of the entire problem, we talked with Peter Pronovost, MD, PhD, one of the country's leading experts on patient safety. Dr. Pronovost is a professor of medicine at the Johns Hopkins University School of Medicine, where he directs the Quality and Safety Research Group. He also serves as the medical director for the Center for Innovation in Quality Care. Dr. Pronovost developed a "checklist" to reduce bloodstream infections. His five-item summary of the most critical infection prevention procedures distilled from the Centers for Disease Control and Prevention guidelines can be used at the bedside. Where the checklist is implemented and enforced and the infection rates are reported, hospital-acquired infections drop significantly.[18] Dr. Pronovost was given a MacArthur "genius" grant in 2009 for his insights and research.

When we interviewed Dr. Pronovost on March 24, 2010, he told us that at least 100,000 people are killed each year by infections they catch in a hospital.[19] He estimated that as many as 100,000 more die from diagnostic errors and suggested that the number may be double that. In addition, Dr. Pronovost counted an additional 50,000 to 100,000 who die from mistakes of commission (medical misadventures). Sins of omission are also significant; he calculated that on average, patients get only about half of the evidence-based therapies they deserve. Such sins would include things like inadequacies in diagnostic testing or not prescribing an essential medication.[20] He admitted that there is no good way to evaluate the harm from these oversights, but he believes deaths from this source may even be more numerous than from any other type of mistakes. He confirmed that [it's] "absolutely right that medical mistakes are the third leading cause of death in America, and the scope of it is frightening. That hasn't really been made public."

These figures don't even include diagnostic mistakes that occur outside hospitals. No one has figured out how to count incorrect diagnoses that are made in doctors' offices, nursing homes, or urgent care clinics. There is reason to believe that these could far outstrip the number of wrong diagnoses that occur in hospitals.

Iatrogenic Deaths

The *Merriam-Webster* online dictionary defines *iatrogenic* as "induced inadvertently by a physician or surgeon or by medical treatment or diagnostic procedures." The total number of deaths that could be considered iatrogenic is difficult to determine. No one organization is counting all the deaths from the various problems that arise in the course of medical care. Pharmacy researchers have attempted to tackle the formidable task of figuring out how many drug-related complications occur outside of hospitals. One study estimated that these account for 199,000 deaths each year.[21]

If you add deaths from medications prescribed in hospitals and nursing homes, the number is far higher. Then there are the deaths caused by misdiagnosis, infections acquired in hospitals or nursing homes, excessive radiation, unnecessary surgery, and postoperative complications. Blood clots resulting from surgical procedures or immobilization in hospital beds account for more than 100,000 deaths annually, and many are preventable. If we add all these figures up, the iatrogenic death toll is over 700,000 a year. This figure exceeds the annual death rate from heart disease or cancer. A great many of these deaths could and should be prevented.

Treatment-Attributable (Iatrogenic) Deaths

Fatal drug reactions (in hospital): 106,000[22] (range is 76,000 to 137,000)

Fatal drug reactions (outpatient): 198,815[23-24]

Fatal drug reactions (nursing homes): 41,652[25-26] (range is 27,768 to 55,535)

Deaths related to misdiagnosis: 132,500[27-30] (range is 40,000 to 225,000)

Health care–acquired infections in hospitals: at least 100,000[31-33]

Deaths from infectious diarrhea in nursing homes: 16,500[34] (These infections are caused by *Clostridium difficile*, a highly infectious and potentially deadly bacteria.)

Excessive radiation from CT (computerized tomography) scans: 29,500[35]

Unnecessary surgery: 12,000[36-37]

Surgical and postoperative complications: 32,591[38-39]

Lethal blood clots in veins (deep vein thrombosis and pulmonary
    embolism): 119,000[40-45] (range is 100,000 to 200,000)

Approximate number of iatrogenic deaths = 788,558

Collateral Damage

Medical screwups can lead to pain and suffering as well as death or
disability. According to the Food and Drug Administration, 1.3 million
people are injured each year by medication mistakes.[46] We have heard
from hundreds of people by mail or e-mail and through comments on
our website. Many have experienced extreme pain and weakness from
their cholesterol-lowering medicine. Often the discomfort gradually
disappears once the medication is discontinued. But there are far too
many situations that change people's lives permanently.

M. described on our website the sad consequences of a screwup during her husband's carotid artery surgery. The doctor came to tell her
that the surgery had been successful, but while they were talking, her
husband nearly died. It took more than twenty minutes to revive him,
and he suffered severe brain damage as a result of that lengthy oxygen
deprivation.

M. was initially told that her husband's heart had just stopped on
its own. But once he was in rehab, she started reviewing his case with
several cardiologists. They concluded, on the basis of tests, that there
was nothing wrong with his heart.

When she finally requested his medical record, she hired an expert
to help her review it. They discovered that the anesthesiologist had removed the breathing tubes and all the monitors in the operating room,
before her husband was moved to the recovery room. When his throat

swelled shut, no one noticed. He was blue and in serious trouble when the staff began reviving him. Since his throat had swelled shut, it was nearly impossible to replace the breathing tube for the oxygen.

M.'s husband had a history of sleep apnea, so the usual procedure would have been to keep him intubated until he was fully awake. Because the anesthesiologist did not follow the appropriate protocol, this fifty-seven-year-old man now has no short-term memory, can't initiate simple tasks, does not speak, and cannot be left alone.

When a patient is harmed as a result of health care, doctors call it an adverse event. Such complications can occur because of a problem in the operating room, as with M.'s husband. Other adverse events may result from reactions to medications. One man became blind in one eye because of a medication called amiodarone (Cordarone, Pacerone) prescribed for atrial fibrillation (an irregular heart rhythm). The drug destroyed his optic nerve. His wife reported on our website that they were not informed of this risk ahead of time and that the doctor insisted upon this drug although it is not the only treatment option.

Treatment-Attributable Adverse Events

• Hospitalized patients with adverse events	45.8 percent[47]
• Outpatients with adverse drug events (ADEs)	18 percent[48] to 25 percent[49]
• Health care–acquired infections	1.7 million[50]
• Annual cost of preventable adverse events	$45.6 billion[51]
• Preventable adverse drug reactions	1.5 million[52]
• Medication mistakes	More than 1/day/ hospital bed[53]
• ICU medication errors	Median 106 per 1,000 patient-days[54]

- Treatable/preventable outpatient adverse drug events (ADE) — 7.8 million[55]
- Percentage of ADEs not addressed by physician — 24 percent[56]
- ADEs in Medicare patients in hospitals (2004) — 888,000[57]
- Adverse events in Medicare patients (2008) — 3.2 million[58]
- Annual cost of medical mistakes — $17 billion to $29 billion[59]

Other adverse events occur when people catch nasty bugs while they are being treated for an unrelated problem. As dangerous as hospitals can be when it comes to spreading deadly infections, they are not the only place where people are exposed. Increasingly, surgery takes place in outpatient ambulatory surgical centers. According to the Ambulatory Surgery Center Association, three-quarters of the operations that take place each year are done in outpatient settings.[60] People go to these facilities for procedures like colonoscopies, cataract surgery, and arthroscopic surgery on knees, shoulders, and other joints. An audit of such facilities showed that many are not following basic infection control guidelines. Two-thirds of the centers studied had "lapses in infection control identified during the inspections."[61]

See No Evil

By any measure, medical errors and adverse drug reactions take a terrible toll. The cost in human terms is incalculable, and the cost in dollars is astronomical. If medical mistakes and misadventures were a disease, there would be a great deal of hand wringing. We would have an organization comparable to the American Heart Association or the American Cancer Society to publicize the problem, and huge sums of tax dollars would be spent researching the causes and seeking solutions to all these screwups. Instead, the medical establishment mostly acts as if this problem were invisible.

The National Cancer Institute has a budget of nearly $5 billion. Nearly half of the money goes for research, and about 10 percent ($472 million) goes to cancer prevention and control. Even though deaths from medications and mistakes account for nearly as many deaths as those from cancer, the safety budget is a pittance. In 2001, Congress allocated $50 million annually for patient safety research, 1 percent of the budget of the National Institutes of Health.[62] Only three years later, funding for patient safety was shifted toward information technology, effectively derailing this critical effort.

Without adequate funding, there is no incentive for hospitals to report errors or implement appropriate safety systems. There is, for example, clear evidence that hospitals can dramatically cut down on infections by following some simple procedures.[63] These include testing every patient who enters a hospital and isolating those with MRSA (methicillin-resistant *Staphylococcus aureus*). Every single staff person who enters such a patient's room must follow strict hand hygiene, gown, glove, and mask precautions. Special cleaning procedures are critical to keep these resistant germs from spreading. All this costs more, but it saves lives as well as money in the long run. Very few hospitals have been willing to spend the initial funds to adopt such proven preventive measures.

Why is it that patient safety is such a low priority? The Institute of Medicine called for a national mandatory reporting system for medical errors in its 1999 report, but more than a decade later, we're no closer to such a system. There was a concerted effort by the American Medical Association and the American Hospital Association to take mandatory public reporting off the table. These groups spent $81 million between 2000 and 2002 lobbying Congress against reporting.[64]

We can only speculate why doctors, hospitals, and pharmacies are so resistant to a national error reporting system. No doubt there is a strong fear of litigation. Physicians and administrators worry that if they fully disclose a mistake, they will be sued, even though the data suggest the opposite.[65] The University of Michigan Health System, for example, implemented a full-disclosure policy in 2001. In addition to telling patients everything that happened, when the hospital investigation determines that an error was made, patients are offered financial compensation. Instead of increasing lawsuits, this transparency program has resulted in lower liability costs.[66] Relatively few other institutions have adopted such a patient-friendly policy of full disclosure and compensation.

Patients' Right to Know

"Patients want to be told about medical errors that occur in their care. Specifically, patients want to be told that an error occurred, how and why the error happened, and what will be done to prevent similar errors in the future; they also want to hear a sincere apology."[67]

Historically there has been a culture of cover-up in medicine.[68] This "wall of silence" has been very effective at keeping mistakes secret.[69] Physicians may also be concerned that revealing so many missteps will result in public outrage. As one expert noted, "Reporting large numbers of adverse events and any serious preventable event brings intense scrutiny from regulators and the public. Thus, most hospitals have relied on spontaneous reporting, which only identifies about 1 in 20 adverse reactions and leads to the perception that injuries from ADRs [adverse drug reactions] are less common than they really are."[70]

Regardless of their reluctance to report mistakes, doctors, nurses, hospitals, pharmacies, and nursing facilities must be accountable for errors. No other profession could get away with so many screwups and still maintain public confidence. When two pilots got distracted and flew one hundred miles past the Minneapolis airport, landing safely but an hour late, they became a laughingstock, and their licenses were revoked, even though no one was hurt. Health care providers may be afraid of shame and similar punishments if the errors they commit became known.

Hear No Evil

The fear of repercussions may be why there has been a strong push in hospitals to adopt a "no-blame" system-oriented approach to uncovering mistakes.[71] The idea was borrowed from the airline industry. Theoretically, removing punishment for reporting errors or "near-miss" events should encourage health care professionals to volunteer information. It's not clear how well this concept is working.

In some settings, technology can reveal problems humans may overlook. For example, many hospitals are now turning to computer-based physician orders (CPOE), which are able to detect and correct some mistakes before they reach patients. Doctors' illegible handwriting, for instance, is no longer a source of prescription mistakes with CPOE.

Some hospitals are also implementing an innovative computerized surveillance system to detect errors or serious drug events based on the orders given to reverse the problem. For example, if a patient on narcotic pain medicine is prescribed naloxone to reverse an overdose, the surveillance system notes this as an error in narcotic dosing. Such automated systems detect errors at a much higher rate than voluntary reporting. In one community hospital, computerized surveillance found twelve times more problems than were voluntarily reported by hospital staff.[72]

Everyone is in favor of improving patient safety, but it's easy to understand why hospital administrators walk on eggs to avoid annoying or alienating doctors. The no-fault approach to detecting medical errors is designed to encourage reporting and avoid scapegoating. But there is increasing concern among leaders of the patient safety movement that the no-blame approach needs to be balanced by requiring accountability from individual health care providers.[73]

One obvious area where providers should be accountable is hand washing.[74] It should be a no-brainer. We know that when doctors or nurses fail to clean their hands adequately between patients, serious infections can spread. Hospitals have installed hand sanitizer dispensers close to patients' rooms. Administrators have admonished clinical staff on the critical importance of hand hygiene. Despite such efforts, in the majority of hospitals, providers wash their hands only 30 to 70 percent of the time they should.[75]

In any other field where lives are at stake, the professional who fails to follow safety guidelines won't last long. That's why commercial pilots always use checklists before they take off. But physicians who don't wash their hands rarely face any consequences. Patient safety experts suggest one strategy: a physician who repeatedly failed to wash his hands would have his clinical privileges revoked for a week and would have to complete two hours of infection control training.[76] These calls for accountability may eventually be employed, but in the meantime it is up to patients and their families to protect themselves from obvious oversights, such as a doctor or nurse approaching without washing hands.

Speak No Evil

No one likes admitting he's made a mistake. And it's only natural to remain silent if we screw up. The old adage "see no evil, hear no evil, speak no evil" is employed far too often. If we get caught, the inclination is to deny, rationalize, or refute.

Doctors, nurses, and pharmacists are just like the rest of us. The inclination to look the other way if a colleague makes a mistake or to remain silent in the face of our own error is human nature. The only difference is that health care providers are dealing with human life; the stakes are much higher than if we bungle our checkbook balance and bounce a check. Doctors have an ethical obligation to report a colleague who puts patients at risk, but they don't always do so. In one survey, a third of those who knew of an impaired or incompetent colleague failed to report him or her to the appropriate authority.[77] The code of silence exists in medicine as it does in law enforcement. This perpetuates risky or unethical behavior.

Physicians and other health care providers are supposed to tell patients and families whenever a mistake is made, even if there is no long-term harm. If someone is injured, or worse yet, killed, there is an absolute obligation to reveal the error. How well do doctors do at coming clean when they blow it? That's a tough question to answer. One group of specialists, pediatricians, has been studied, and the answers are shocking. In one survey, 439 pediatric attending physicians and 118 residents responded anonymously to a questionnaire. Almost all of them (99 percent) agreed that serious errors should be reported to patients' families.[78] In addition, 90 percent thought that a minor mistake should be acknowledged.

It is refreshing that pediatricians are so committed to the idea of transparency. But how well would they do if put to the test? In another study, pediatricians were surveyed about how they would handle a hypothetical scenario.[79] Half of them were asked about a mistake that would be apparent to the family and half about a mistake that would not be obvious. Nearly three-quarters of the pediatricians would tell parents if the mistake would be obvious. One-third would have offered an explicit apology. In contrast, if the error would be less apparent, only one-third would tell the child's family, and one-fifth would offer an explicit apology.

Pediatricians Study Scenarios

- In the first hypothetical case, pediatricians were asked how they would respond if they administered too much insulin to a child who then had to be admitted to the intensive care unit. This is an obvious mistake.

- In the second hypothetical case, pediatricians were asked how they would respond if they failed to follow up on a laboratory test that showed a child had an infection. The child subsequently developed symptoms and had to be admitted to the hospital. This mistake would be less obvious to the parents.

The authors concluded that "framing the decision to disclose an error based on whether the patient or family is aware of the error is in conflict with standards established by the Joint Commission on Accreditation of Healthcare Organizations and raises challenging ethical questions regarding truth-telling in medicine."[80] If one can generalize from this research, it is clear that in many instances physicians do not openly admit their mistakes to patients or their families. This is despite a clear mandate from the national hospital accrediting body "that all unanticipated outcomes of care be disclosed."[81-82]

When Joe's mother, Helen, died, we were intially told that she fell on the way to the bathroom and died. It was only weeks afterward that we were able to review the records and piece together all the errors that contributed to her unnecessary death. Not all families can make sense of medical records, but all want acknowledgment of mistakes and an apology. Perhaps most important, they want changes instituted that will protect others from experiencing a similar mishap.

Patients are not stupid. They often know when something bad has happened, whether the error is officially disclosed or not. In one study, more than 600 patients were surveyed after their hospital discharge.[83] They reported that they had experienced a total of 845 adverse events, which were verified by the researchers. Unfortunately, only 40 percent of these problems were disclosed to the patients at the time. If providers thought the error was less obvious to the patient, they were much less likely to reveal it. Interestingly, patients who said the mistake had been discussed with them gave a higher rating of the quality of their care.

If you suspect a serious screwup, the chances are pretty good that you are right. Do not assume that you will always be told the truth automatically. Ask! If you are unsatisfied with the answer, request your medical records. You can also ask to speak with someone in authority at the hospital. When in doubt, go straight to the chief medical officer or the chief executive officer (CEO). That is more likely to get results than just about anything else you try.

Top 10 Tips to Stopping Screwups in Hospitals

Faced with the risk of so many potential errors and so little transparency, what's a patient or family to do? Remember that the highly regarded Institute of Medicine report concluded that there are at least 1.5 million preventable adverse drug events that occur in hospitals and long-term care facilities each year. The authors of the report actually believe that "the true number may be much higher."[84] That translates to at least one medication error per patient per day.[85] Other types of errors, from diagnostic mistakes and misplaced lab results to lapses in hygiene and oversights during transitions, also cause uncounted problems. We can only conclude that not experiencing errors while in a hospital would be unusual. We have come up with our own checklist to try to help you from becoming a negative statistic.

• **Number one: Expect mistakes.** Anticipate that there will be missteps every day you or a friend or loved one is in the hospital. Some may be trivial, such as the wrong kind of food on the dinner tray. Others are life threatening, like the wrong medicine in the IV (intravenous line). It is crucial for the hospitalized person to have someone with her at all times. If the patient cannot speak up, ask questions, and verify virtually everything that is done; the advocate must step in and take charge. The patient's life may depend upon the advocate's vigilance.

• **Number two: Drug-check!** Ask about every medicine that is administered and make sure the dose has been calculated correctly. Even though you may not know how to pronounce the drug names or determine the correct dose yourself, just asking the nurse, pharmacist, or physician to verify that all is right can help catch some errors. Make sure someone has checked for drug incompatibility, since hospitalized patients often receive multiple medicines that might interact. Also confirm that the medication about to be administered is truly meant for this patient. Bar-coded wrist bands are used in some hospitals to match up with bar-coded medications. Whoever administers the medications should always double-check the bar codes. And whenever you pick up a prescription at your local pharmacy, double-check to make sure you have the right medicine in the right dose before you leave! Mistakes are far more common than you would ever imagine possible. One study found roughly 4 errors a day in an average pharmacy filling 250 prescriptions. That translates to more than 50 million errors a year across the country.[86]

• **Number three: Be assertive!** Don't be afraid to be difficult. Patients, friends, and family members may worry that asking hard questions about drugs, lab results, and procedures may give the patient in room 309 a reputation for being troublesome. The fear is that this could lead to less attentive care. But the squeaky wheel gets the grease. Hospital staff may find the questions annoying and time consuming, but they will adapt to answering them and double-checking. Being nice can get you killed.

Mother as Advocate

"My daughter had complex medical problems and was hospitalized many times at a prominent children's hospital. There was at least one medication error during every stay. My daughter was disabled, so I stayed with her while she was in the hospital and always checked her medications carefully. This avoided many potential errors.

"She also had a latex allergy. I examined every item that entered her room to make sure there was no latex. Had it not been for my vigilance, she could well have suffered anaphylactic shock.

"Eventually her chart was flagged, and the nursing supervisor visited her room frequently to make sure everything was going smoothly. I still worry about children who are alone in the hospital. They may get medications that might not be the correct ones."

• **Number four: Say no!** When in doubt, object. Every patient has the right to say no, decline a medicine or a procedure, or even leave the hospital. If you suspect that a medicine is incorrect or that a procedure is inappropriate, you can and should refuse. Going along just to be a "good patient" could cause irreparable harm. "NO!" gets everyone's attention very quickly. It's a little like a monkey wrench in the machinery of the hospital. If you demand an explanation from an attending physician, you will eventually get one. Then the machinery can start working again.

• **Number five: Track transitions.** Hospitals refer to them as handoffs. Whenever things or people change, there are greater chances for screwups. When you move from the emergency room into a hospital bed, not all the relevant information may travel with you. The same is true whenever you leave the room for a procedure or test. Shift changes, when the night nursing staff goes off duty and is replaced by the day nurses, is another opportunity for vital information to get lost. Make sure your advocate is on hand for these transitions so that he or she is included in the team handover conversation and can be informed of your status.

• **Number six: Call "Condition H" (Help).** If a friend or family member suspects that something bad is happening, that person should immediately alert the nursing staff. If the reaction is not satisfactory, ask for a rapid response team to be sent. Many hospitals now have a special team of experts who react promptly to a "Condition H" call and assess the patient's situation to determine if special action should be taken.

• **Number seven: Deal with discharge.** When you leave the hospital, be sure to get detailed instructions and contact information. Everyone wants to get home as quickly as possible, but the discharge process can be an opportunity for disaster. Know what symptoms might signal a worsening situation or a hospital-acquired infection. Find out what to do and whom to call if anything seems out of line. Get specific instructions on the medicines you are supposed to take, how to take them, and what the most common or serious side effects may be. Ask if your medical records can be sent to you so you can share them with your doctor. They are legally yours, though the institution may charge a copying fee.

• **Number eight: Cultivate communication.** Do not assume that your doctors have spoken to one another. There is a very good chance that your hospital doctors will never speak with your primary care provider. So it behooves you to take your medical records and notes along to your next visit so you can bring the nurse practitioner or family practice doctor up to date on what you have been through, complete with all the diagnoses, procedures, and medications. In most cases, the primary care provider will be the one who follows up and helps you with your recovery. Even if you have not been hospitalized, don't assume that the cardiologist you saw last month has made a full report to the internist or the urologist you may be seeing today. You need to be able to summarize the relevant information so that nothing gets overlooked. It will be helpful for you to keep information with you, whether in print or electronically, to share with all your providers.

• **Number nine: Double-check everything.** Whenever you have any lab work done or diagnostic procedures carried out, make sure you get a copy of the results in a timely fashion. Do not assume that no news is good news. Doctors sometimes do not see your lab results because they get buried under piles of paper and ignored. Or the physician may simply get distracted and forget to notify you, even if the result is not normal.[87] In some practices, this oversight happens one time out of four times. And do not always assume the results are correct. Pathology reports, X-rays, or blood work can be inaccurate. If something seems out of line, don't hesitate to ask for a repeat test, since you may have gotten Mr. Smith's results by accident. You don't want your doctor to treat you based on faulty information.

• **Number ten: Take a friend or family member.** Nearly all the mistakes that can be made in hospitals also occur in an outpatient setting. That includes misdiagnoses, poor hand hygiene and infection control, and errors in prescribing medicine or calculating a dose. Just as you need an advocate in the hospital, you should also take a family member or friend along whenever you are getting health care. A second pair of eyes and ears can be very useful in getting instructions and spotting problems. To get the most from a doctor visit, many people find it helpful to prepare a checklist ahead of time with questions and concerns in order of priority (most important first!). If you have problems and suspect they may be related to your medication, don't assume the provider can read your mind. Speak up and let her know what is going on, and then make sure she takes action. It may be up to you to follow up if the course of action does not fully resolve the problem.

CHAPTER 2

TOP 10 SCREWUPS DOCTORS MAKE

1. Not listening to patients
2. Misdiagnosing
3. Providing too little information
4. Not dealing with side effects
5. Undertreating or ignoring the evidence
6. Overreacting or being seduced by numbers
7. Overlooking drug interactions
8. Failing to revise the plan
9. Overlooking lab results
10. Not addressing lifestyle issues

Top 10 lists focus the mind. They force us to prioritize. Of course, they risk oversimplifying a complex problem. We recognize that an enormous number of mistakes are made in health care and that trying to boil them down to the top 10 is risky business. Nevertheless, we hope you will consider the lists that follow in the spirit in which they are intended: to help you avoid experiencing a mistake that could lead to harm. We could not cover all the issues, but we did want to focus on what we believe are the really big potholes on the path to good outcomes.

Doctors have an impossible job. They have to learn way more information than any human is capable of retaining during their medical school education and residency training. Then they have to keep up with the latest developments in research and treatment despite grueling hours seeing patients. They frequently have to wrestle with insurance companies and all sorts of other bureaucratic bottlenecks. Finally, they are under enormous time pressure to see as many patients as possible. We have talked with many doctors who complain about having to practice "assembly line medicine." It's no wonder that sometimes doctors make mistakes. Here are our top 10 to watch out for.

Top 10 Doctor Screwups

• **Number one: Not listening to patients.** Studies repeatedly show that many doctors have a habit of interrupting patients within twelve to twenty seconds of the beginning of an office visit.[1-4] This frequently means that the patient never gets to tell the whole story. When sidetracked by an interruption, she may not ever get to finish telling the doctor about her chief concerns. Because a proper diagnosis depends so much on the patient's story, interruptions interfere with the ability to make the right diagnosis and determine the best course of treatment.

In his book *How Doctors Think,* Dr. Jerome Groopman describes a doctor's diagnostic effort as "thought-in-action," with the doctor coming up with his most likely two or three diagnoses while he says hello and begins the physical exam or looks at test results.[5] The shortcuts doctors use help them get to the proper diagnosis promptly at least some of the time, but they can also lead to screwups unless the doctor is also intently listening to the patient. Be assertive, and make sure your entire story is heard and understood. Ask your doctor to tell you what he heard so you can verify that he really got it.

• **Number two: Misdiagnosing.** One of the primary reasons to visit a physician or go to a hospital is to find out what's wrong. We assume that all those arduous years of training have prepared doctors to figure out exactly why we are having symptoms. It turns out that misdiagnosis is far more common than most patients ever imagine. In their groundbreaking article in the *Journal of the American Medical Association,* "Diagnostic Errors—The Next Frontier for Patient Safety," David Newman-Toker, MD, PhD, and Peter Pronovost, MD, PhD, revealed shocking statistics.[6] They stated that "an estimated 40,000 to 80,000 US hospital deaths result from misdiagnosis annually."[7] Later, during a radio interview with us, they confided that it is probably more than 100,000 deaths in hospitals each year.[8] Dr. Newman-Toker admitted that "this could be the tip of the iceberg. We really don't know, and we won't know until we have better measurement techniques to assess just how frequent missed diagnoses are." If you include diagnostic errors for outpatients, the numbers are staggering.

Pancreatitis Puzzle

"Several years ago, I developed severe stomach pains and vomiting shortly after arriving at work. I went to an urgent care clinic, where a doctor told me it was probably severe acid reflux and sent me on my way with Prevacid.

"A couple of hours later, the pain was much worse. A friend took me to the trauma center of the same hospital, and I passed out before being seen.

"After numerous tests that took several days, the doctors determined that I had acute pancreatitis. I also had undiagnosed severe type 2 diabetes (blood glucose of 350) and hyperlipidemia (6,600). My husband spent days fighting with the docs to convince them that I was not an alcoholic. Tests finally proved that, too.

"While in the hospital, I developed a staph infection through a central line. The pancreas became necrotic and required twelve surgeries, one every other day. I was put in a coma to recover. It took me six weeks of inpatient rehab before I could do even the simplest of things."

• **Number three: Providing too little information.** Physicians are placed in an untenable position. On the one hand, they are told to follow the tenets of the Hippocratic oath, which includes the admonition to "do no harm." On the other hand, every medicine they prescribe has the potential to cause side effects, at least in some people. This double bind often results in doctors' glossing over possible side effects for fear that mentioning them will bring them on by the power of suggestion. But not telling the patient of common or serious complications of a therapy can have devastating consequences.

Research has shown that "most patients want more information than physicians usually give. . . . To do this, the physician must ask the patient what he or she wants to know. The physician must also confirm with patients that they have understood what was said."[9] This is crucial every time a physician and patient interact, especially during an emergency. Nevertheless, in one study of emergency room doctors, researchers found that "information on diagnosis, expected course of illness, self-care, use of medications, time-specified follow-up, and symptoms that should prompt return to the ED [emergency department] were each discussed less than 65 percent of the time. Only 16 percent of patients were asked whether they had questions, and there were no instances in which the provider confirmed patient understanding of the information."[10]

The "teach-back" technique calls for a doctor to ask the patient what he or she has heard to verify that the communication was clear. This is also a useful technique for patients to make sure that the doctor has registered their symptoms and concerns.

• **Number four: Not dealing with side effects.** This one is mind blowing. You would think that if patients reported side effects from a medicine, most physicians would respond promptly to try to solve the problem. But at least one study showed that doctors failed to address one out of four patient-reported symptoms.[11] The authors concluded that "extrapolating to the 98.9 million annual visits to US internists by patients who received a medication or for whom a medication was prescribed during the visit, as many as 7.8 million ADEs [adverse drug events] could be prevented or ameliorated if patients and their physicians communicated better and if physicians acted more reliably to address medication symptoms."[12]

We are amazed. How can physicians ignore drug-induced side effects 25 percent of the time? We wouldn't believe it if we didn't hear about it so often. One drug in particular demonstrates this discouraging oversight better than any other.

No one gets out of medical school without learning about a class of blood pressure medications called ACE (angiotensin-converting enzyme) inhibitors. These are among the most commonly prescribed drugs in the pharmacy. Roughly 100 million prescriptions are filled each year for such medicines, and lisinopril (Prinivil, Zestril) is by far the most popular. One of the most common side effects of all these medications is a cough, affecting up to one-third of those taking such drugs.

Cough medicine won't stop this cough. The only solution is to switch to a completely different kind of blood pressure drug. This is as basic as it gets. We continue to be astonished that so many people have posted to our website that their physicians did not recognize that their cough was caused by an ACE inhibitor like lisinopril or ramipril (Altace). That is like banging your thumb with a hammer and wondering why it hurts and why the nail turns black. What really worries us, though, is that if some physicians can't connect the dots when it comes to lisinopril and cough, what other drug-induced side effects are they missing?

Drug-induced Cough

"I started taking lisinopril for high blood pressure. Soon I developed a nagging dry cough that I couldn't shake. I have thrown up because the coughing was so bad. I have had blood tests and chest X-rays that all came back negative.

"In desperation, I went to an ENT [ear, nose and throat] specialist, who told me this kind of cough is common in people my age (fifty) due to post-nasal drip. He knew I was on lisinopril, but he gave me an antihistamine and cough suppressant. Of course, they didn't help.

"I learned on your website that lisinopril can cause a chronic cough. I am furious that none of the doctors I've seen warned me or suggested changing this medicine."

• **Number five: Undertreating or ignoring the evidence.** Doctors have adopted a mantra called "evidence-based medicine." The idea behind it is to use treatments that have been proved effective. Dr. Pronovost has suggested that far too many patients die because their physicians failed to implement the best treatment for their condition.

One of the most obvious examples is a failure to prescribe an inexpensive generic drug called spironolactone (Aldactone) for patients with congestive heart failure (CHF), a common and very dangerous condition in which the heart has trouble pumping blood efficiently. Nearly 6 million Americans suffer from congestive heart failure, and one out of five dies within the first year after diagnosis.[13] Spironolactone is thought of as a treatment for hypertension, though it also helps with fluid retention, a serious complication of CHF. A study in 1999 showed that spironolactone saved lives.[14] An editorial in the *New England Journal of Medicine* reinforced the ability of this inexpensive diuretic to improve heart function.[15] The American Heart Association started a "Get with the Guidelines" program to encourage the use of spironolactone in heart failure patients. Nonetheless, ten years after the original study, only one-third of heart failure patients in 201 hospitals had been prescribed this medication.[16] That means two-thirds did not receive optimal treatment. What other professional could ignore guidelines or best practices so routinely and not be chastised?

It's hard for patients and their families to know what the best choices are for treating a specific condition. One place to look online is the Cochrane Collaboration (www.cochrane.org). Health experts from around the world volunteer to evaluate what works (including alternative therapies) for various conditions. Our book *Best Choices from the People's Pharmacy* is another resource.

• **Number six: Overtreating or being seduced by numbers.** Doctors who don't understand how to evaluate statistics regarding drug effectiveness may easily fall prey to drug company advertising. These ads often lead them to overestimate benefits and underestimate risks. Many doctors believe that more is better. We have another phrase for this idea, the "lottle" principle: if a little is good, then a lottle will be better. We see this frequently with cholesterol control. There was a time when getting total cholesterol under 220 mg/dL and bad LDL (low-density lipoprotein) cholesterol under 135 mg/dL was considered acceptable. Then the bar was set lower (total cholesterol under 200 and LDL cholesterol under 100). Now doctors frequently prescribe high doses of a statin-type cholesterol-lowering drug plus one or two other medications to get total cholesterol under 180 and LDL cholesterol under 70. Those numbers are only appropriate if a patient has serious heart disease. Expert analysts for the Cochrane Collaboration reviewed data from fourteen studies involving more than 30,000 subjects. They reported in 2011 that there was "limited evidence" that statins extend or improve life for people without clear signs of heart disease.[17] Three-quarters of the people who are prescribed statins are just such healthy people.[18]

Diabetes is an even more compelling example. Doctors treating type 2 diabetes often try hard to get their patients' blood sugar as close to normal as possible. This is called "tight control." The goal is to reduce the risk of heart attacks, strokes, kidney disease, and other complications of diabetes. It seemed like such a good idea. But a large, long-term trial called ACCORD (Action to Control Cardiovascular Risk in Diabetes) stunned the medical community. Aggressive treatment of blood sugar in these patients resulted in more heart attacks and deaths rather than fewer.[19] Intensive treatment of blood pressure to get systolic pressure down to 120 or less did not reduce the rate of heart attack or death significantly.[20] Not surprisingly, serious adverse reactions were substantially more common among those who got intensive treatment.

Another part of the ACCORD trial examined aggressive control of lipids (LDL cholesterol and triglycerides) in people with diabetes. There was another surprise. Adding the drug fenofibrate (TriCor) to simvastatin (Zocor) did not affect the risk of heart attack, stroke, or death.[21] That said, commercials for a medication similar to Tricor called Trilipix encourage patients to "ask your doctor" to consider adding this medication to a statin for extra protection, even though there are no data to suggest that doing so would reduce the risk of heart attacks or strokes. The ads are working, since doctors prescribe Trilipix and Tricor in substantial quantities, frequently in combination with statins.

• **Number seven: Overlooking drug interactions.** We have been writing about the dangers of drug interactions for more than thirty-five years. This is truly one of the colossal screwups that doctors make on a regular basis, and it accounts for an astonishing amount of disability and death. It is ironic and incredibly painful to know that a drug interaction directly contributed to Joe's mother's death.

Americans take an astonishing number of medications, and not all of them get along. Researchers have found that 81 percent of older adults took prescribed drugs. More than half "used 5 or more prescription medications, over-the-counter medications, or dietary supplements."[22] A surprising number of people swallow dozens of pills daily.

There are so many potentially dangerous drug interactions that no human can possibly remember even a fraction of them. As a result, every time a medication is prescribed, possible incompatibilities with other medicines, vitamins, herbs, or dietary supplements should be taken into consideration. We suspect it is rare for a busy prescriber to take the time to do this. Even when the doctor has a sophisticated electronic prescribing system that warns him about dangerous drug interactions before the prescription can be entered, it's not unusual for the clinician to decide to override the alert and prescribe the drug anyway. In one study, prescribers ignored more than half of these alerts, even for potentially serious interactions.[23]

A fascinating study was conducted to test prescribers' knowledge of potential drug-drug interactions. Questionnaires were mailed to 12,500 physicians, nurse practitioners, and physician assistants. These prescribers were asked to determine the safety of fourteen drug pairings. Of the 950 who responded, fewer than half correctly identified all the unsafe combinations. Because this was a "take-home" test, these health professionals could have looked up the answers on their computers or in a reference book, though they were asked to restrict use of drug references when answering. Four out of five prescribers did not recognize the danger of combining the acid reducer cimetidine (Tagamet) with the blood thinner warfarin (Coumadin). Such a combination could cause a serious hemorrhage. The researchers concluded that "this study suggests that prescribers' knowledge of potential clinically significant DDIs [drug-drug interactions] is generally poor."[24]

The researchers discovered that physicians frequently learned about dangerous combinations from pharmacists. But even when pharmacists detect a serious drug interaction, they aren't always able to get in touch with the prescriber. Pharmacists have confided to us that many physicians do not return their calls promptly, if at all.

• **Number eight: Failing to revise the plan.** A popular definition of insanity is "doing the same thing over and over again and expecting different results." We frequently hear from patients who have experienced severe muscle pain and weakness as a side effect of a statin-type cholesterol-lowering drug. The doctor responds by prescribing another statin. Although this occasionally works, more often than not the patient has the same symptoms all over again, only to be prescribed yet a different statin.

The same type of thing happens with people who can't tolerate antidepressant medications like fluoxetine (Prozac) or sertraline (Zoloft). If the doctor prescribes a drug in the same general category such as paroxetine (Paxil) or venlafaxine (Effexor), symptoms such as sexual difficulties, nausea, headache, or dizziness are likely to persist.

In his book *Safe Patients, Smart Hospitals,* Dr. Pronovost tells about a patient who was not doing well after surgery. The surgeon refused to have the patient admitted to intensive care because he was adamant that he had done nothing wrong during the surgery. The woman would have died if Dr. Pronovost had not intervened and changed the surgeon's postop care plan. As it was, she lost a previously healthy kidney and suffered grievous harm because of the surgeon's intransigence.[25]

• **Number nine: Overlooking lab results.** In a busy practice, a doctor orders a lot of lab tests for diagnosis or monitoring. Unless she has a well-organized system in place for tracking the results when they come back, important information may fall through the cracks. This is far more common than most people realize. Researchers reviewed medical records of over 5,000 patients in twenty-three different medical practices. The investigators discovered more than 1,800 abnormal test results. Of these, 135 patients had never been told the results of their test. That means 1 out of 14 patients with abnormal results did not hear about them.[26] Practices varied enormously in their failure rates. In some cases, as many as one-quarter of abnormal test results were not communicated to the patient. In other practices, every worrisome lab finding was relayed to the patient.

Not communicating test results to a patient can be life threatening. If a mammogram shows something suspicious, but that information is not given to the patient, a year or more may pass before a proper diagnosis is made and the breast cancer treated. If blood sugar levels start creeping up, a person could end up with full-blown diabetes that could have been treated earlier. The lesson for the patient is never to assume that no news is good news. Always follow up with a doctor who has ordered any test or procedure. If you have not heard within a week or two, contact the office and insist on learning your results.

• **Number ten: Not addressing lifestyle issues.** Doctors know that healthy habits could replace a lot of medication. Researchers have proved this beyond a shadow of a doubt. One study from Britain followed almost 5,000 adults for about twenty years. People with poor health habits (smoking, drinking too much, not exercising, and eating badly) were likely to die twelve years earlier on average.[27]

Even though physicians frequently tell their patients to lose weight, stop smoking, and exercise more, everyone gets frustrated at the lack of progress. Most doctors don't know *how* to help patients change their behavior; teaching those skills is not a priority in medical school. That means primary care providers don't have the tools to coach their patients in adopting and maintaining healthy lifestyles, and in fact they often don't see it as their responsibility. Eric Westman, MD, director of the Duke Lifestyle Medicine Clinic, points out that doctors learn how to prescribe pills, not how to help people lose weight and keep it off.[28] In addition, physicians are not held accountable for their patients' weight gain, even when medicines they prescribe are known to cause substantial weight gain as a side effect.

Don't look to your doctor for a lot of help when it comes to healthy habits. A wellness coach might be far more helpful. Such people understand behavior, motivation, and coaching strategies that can keep you making progress.

CHAPTER 3

DIAGNOSTIC DISASTERS

Diagnosis is the key to successful medical treatment. Before any drug can be prescribed, surgical procedure initiated, or any other action taken, the doctor must have a pretty good idea of what's going on with a patient. Physicians like to think of themselves as well grounded in science. Unlike their forefathers, who often depended on instinct and experience, today's medical doctors believe they rely on evidence to make decisions. In fact the phrase "evidence-based medicine" has become a mantra that means modern practitioners are supposed to rely far more on logic, data, and technology than intuition.

Scientists or Gamblers?

Here's a little secret that most physicians have a hard time admitting: they are gamblers as much as scientists. That is to say, they play the odds. It sounds better if we say physicians use statistics and probabilities when diagnosing, but it is basically the same thing.

It all starts in medical school with another favorite phrase: "When you hear hoofbeats, think horses, not zebras." What that means is that medical students, interns, and residents are taught to look for the most obvious diagnosis—that is, a horse rather than something rare or exotic, like a zebra. Another way of describing this concept is "Ockham's razor," extolled by the English logician William of Ockham in the fourteenth century. This "principle of parsimony" teaches that when there are various possibilities for solving a problem, the simplest is usually the best.

This is the kind of logic that poker players employ. Someone playing Texas hold'em who is dealt an ace of hearts and an ace of spades predicts that he has a very good chance of winning against his opponent.

If the other player has a seven of hearts and a four of spades the actual odds would be 85.16 percent to 14.36 percent. The man with the aces will stay in the game and probably raise whenever possible. The fellow with the crappy hand should fold because that is the most obvious way to play the odds. But as every poker player knows, sometimes you get dealt unpredictable cards. The guy with the aces may not see another good card, while the fellow with the seven and four could get a five, a six, and an eight, giving him a straight and the winning hand.

That is the lure of poker. You can play the odds and win a lot of the time, but not infrequently you lose. The same thing happens in medicine. Sometimes what seems like an obvious diagnosis turns out to be wrong. The difference between poker and medicine is that if the doctor loses the bet, you could suffer or die.[1]

Tick Fever

"I told doctors at an urgent care facility, then my internist, then a doctor in the emergency room, and, during my hospital stay, three infectious disease specialists that I believed I may have been bitten by a tick. All refused to believe there could be a tick bite in Georgia in late December. They never tested me for tick-borne fevers despite my request.

"I was very ill, running a fever as high as 107 with complications. I had a lengthy hospital stay and a recovery time of months, all because no one would address my tick bite concerns and simply give me a four-dollar prescription for doxycycline as a precaution.

"It was only because the hospital lab sent my blood to the state health department based on my continued tick bite concerns that my blood was tested for tick-borne fevers and a diagnosis of ehrlichiosis was confirmed."

R. H.

It turns out that although the odds of getting a tick bite are lower in winter, they are not zero. If the temperature gets above 35 degrees Fahrenheit for several days (quite possible in Georgia in late December), ticks can rouse themselves and start looking for food (a blood meal). Ehrlichiosis is a tick-borne disease that resembles the flu (mild fever, fatigue, headache, and cough). Untreated, this disease can lead to very high fever, seizures, or even kidney failure.

The probability approach to diagnosis is understandable, especially when time is money. The faster the diagnosis, the more quickly a patient can be given a prescription and sent on his way. When a physician has a waiting room full of patients, it is far more efficient to proceed as if you are dealing with a horse than a zebra, which could take a lot longer to corral. And much of the time it works.

Unfortunately, some conditions that doctors often think of as zebras are actually much more common. One of the biggest mistakes with regard to celiac disease, for example, is considering it a rare condition. For decades, medical students were taught that this autoimmune disorder would show up in only 1 case out of 5,000 patients. But better research now reveals that celiac disease is far more common, affecting approximately 1 American in every 133.[2] This is partly because the disease, an inflammatory response to gluten (a protein found in wheat, barley, and rye) that occurs in some genetically susceptible people, has actually become more frequent in the last fifty years,[3] and partly because earlier doctors weren't looking for it.

Celiac disease is easy to miss because the symptoms can be so variable and nonspecific. Many people who are diagnosed with irritable bowel syndrome are later found to have celiac disease. Undiagnosed celiac disease can cause a lot of suffering and increase the risk of premature death, so it is prudent for a doctor to include it in the list of possible problems when considering a diagnosis.

Gluten Illness

"I suffered from abdominal pain, gas, bloating, constipation, and diarrhea as well as joint pain for over ten years. Three different doctors told me that I suffered from irritable bowel syndrome, with symptoms mild enough to be controlled with over-the-counter drugs, meditation, and other stress reduction techniques.

"My last physician told me that she suspected rheumatoid arthritis because of the joint pain. If it continued for a few more months, she'd put me on steroids. At age thirty!

"I specifically asked if these problems could be food related, and no one thought they were. Finally I was bedridden four days out of seven with severe abdominal pain and woke each morning with knees so stiff and sore that walking was a chore for the first ten minutes of the day. I consulted a naturopathic doctor, who discovered I am sensitive to gluten. Within three days of cutting wheat from my diet, I was a new woman, with no joint or abdominal pain!"

Misdiagnoses: A Silent Epidemic

The trouble with looking for the obvious diagnosis is that it leads to mistakes. And diagnostic mistakes there are aplenty. This may well be the biggest secret in medicine. Until very recently, diagnostic errors weren't even studied. No one was bold enough to really start asking hard questions or seeking answers. No one, that is, until Peter Pronovost, MD, PhD, and David Newman-Toker, MD, PhD, wrote their 2009 landmark commentary in the *Journal of the American Medical Association*: "Diagnostic Errors—The Next Frontier for Patient Safety."[4]

These two patient safety experts revealed some amazing truths. Here are some selected quotes:

- "Diagnostic errors have received relatively little attention."
- "An estimated 40,000 to 80,000 U.S. hospital deaths result from misdiagnosis annually. Roughly 5 percent of autopsies reveal lethal diagnostic errors for which a correct diagnosis coupled with treatment could have averted death."
- "Diagnostic errors often are unrecognized or unreported, and the science of measuring these errors (and their effects) is underdeveloped."
- "According to a recent systematic review, 9 percent of all cerebrovascular events [strokes] are missed initially, and the odds of misdiagnosis increases at least 5-fold when symptoms are mild or transient. Thus, misdiagnoses probably represent an enormous unmeasured source of preventable mortality, morbidity, and costs."

Surprisingly, the response from the medical community to this incredible article has been a big yawn. The reaction to the 1999 IOM report "To Err Is Human" was overwhelming.[5] There have been thousands of articles written about this problem. Diagnostic errors, on the other hand, have been neglected.[6] Even though they account for twice as many medical malpractice suits as any other kind of mistake, they are rarely studied and get no respect.[7]

If anything, Drs. Pronovost and Newman-Toker erred on the side of caution in their *JAMA* commentary. When last we spoke with Dr. Pronovost, he told us that misdiagnoses in hospitals may actually lead to 100,000 deaths annually,[8] and a more recent report suggests that the number may be double that. These two patient safety experts based their estimates in part on an autopsy-identified error rate of 5 percent. Other researchers have noted that "errors related to delayed or missed diagnoses are a frequent and underappreciated cause of patient injury. While the exact prevalence of diagnostic error remains unknown, data from autopsy series spanning several decades conservatively and consistently reveal error rates of 10 percent to 15 percent."[9]

Even those numbers may be low. Several years ago the *New York Times* reported that "studies of autopsies have shown that doctors seriously misdiagnose fatal illnesses about 20 percent of the time. So millions of patients are being treated for the wrong disease."[10] In 1998, George Lundberg, MD, then editor-in-chief of the *Journal of the American Medical Association,* wrote that "diagnostic discordance" had been noted since the 1930s. He observed that over the next six decades approximately 40 percent of the time the diagnosis that was made before death was different from that revealed by the autopsy.[11] If anything, the problem seemed to be getting worse. Dr. Lundberg's damning indictment: "No improvement!" What's more, in one study two-thirds of the missed diagnoses were for conditions that could have been successfully treated.[12]

- Experts who have analyzed all the available data conclude that diagnostic error rates in clinical medicine can be as high as 15 percent.[13-14] The bottom line seems to be that diagnostic errors are the elephant in the room that most doctors do not want to talk about and don't know how to fix.

Common Diagnostic Mistakes

When given the opportunity to discuss this issue anonymously, however, doctors reveal some fascinating facts. Researchers surveyed 310 clinicians (internists, medical specialists, and emergency room docs) at twenty-two institutions. They asked their colleagues to "report 3 cases of diagnostic errors and to describe their perceived causes, seriousness, and frequency. . . . Our collection of anonymous cases and descriptions of 'what went wrong' and 'why did it happen' afforded those committing an error the opportunity to candidly share (or, in the words of several respondents, 'to confess') errors in a blame-free context."[15] Of the 533 physician-reported cases, here are the most frequently missed diagnoses in descending order:

Top 10 Diagnostic Screwups[16]

1. Pulmonary embolism (blood clot in lungs)

2. Drug reaction or overdose

3. Lung cancer

4. Colorectal cancer

5. Acute coronary syndrome (including heart attack)

6. Breast cancer

7. Strokes

8. Congestive heart failure

9. Fractures, various types

10. Abscesses

Other diagnostic errors reported by this group of physicians were associated with pneumonia, aortic aneurysm, appendicitis, depression, and diabetes. This was not a particularly scientific study. It relied on the participants' memory, and there was no review of medical records to confirm mistakes. Nevertheless, the study revealed "patterns of errors." What is so fascinating about the top 10 diagnostic screwups reported by this relatively small group of physicians is that it mirrors the problems that show up in large databases of malpractice claims.

If you want to know what conditions are most often misdiagnosed and lead to harm, ask malpractice insurance companies. These organizations have to defend physicians, clinics, and hospitals when they are sued. Insurance companies keep careful records of claims. When you review the data, you find surprising overlap with the kinds of conditions the doctors self-reported above.[17-19]

Common Diagnostic Screwups
Leading to Malpractice Claims

- Cancers (lung, breast, colorectal)
- Fractures
- Infections
- Pulmonary embolism (blood clot in lungs)
- Heart attacks
- Strokes
- Appendicitis
- Diabetes

Is there any other profession that would accept an error rate of 15 percent as normal? Who would put up with an accountant who screwed up their tax return on a regular basis? If pilots landed planes at the wrong destination one out of seven times, there would be a hue and cry, and immediate action would be taken to correct the problem. And yet the medical profession has tolerated an unacceptable diagnostic error rate for decades, and no one has said boo.

It is time for medicine to be as accountable as any other profession. Researchers are beginning to realize that there is a huge problem with diagnostic errors. Not only do diagnostic errors have to be studied so that we can better understand where the problems are, but we have to figure out ways to stop many of them from happening. If millions of people are misdiagnosed every year, that means that many are being treated for the wrong condition. It is not okay to accept so many mistakes as normal.

CHAPTER 4

TOP 10 REASONS WHY
DOCTORS SCREW UP DIAGNOSES

1. Overconfidence
2. Information overload
3. Going it alone
4. Tunnel vision
5. Time pressure
6. Missing test results
7. Ignoring drug side effects
8. Follow-up failure
9. Hurried hand-offs
10. Communication breakdown

How is it possible that such smart people, who have been trained so intensely for so long, make so many diagnostic errors? Training is a big part of the problem. In fact, it starts even before the training begins. Medical students are selected for their extraordinary ability to memorize and regurgitate huge amounts of information. On the surface, that might seem like a good thing, but in truth it reinforces the idea that it is possible to memorize everything that you need to know to practice medicine.

Setting Doctors Up for Diagnostic Failures

Charlie Burger, MD, a doc in Bangor, Maine, who has been practicing his craft since 1971, summed up the problem in an interview with the *Bangor Daily News*:

" 'All of medical education is geared toward cramming as much information as possible into our heads,' on the unrealistic assumption that doctors will be able to recall the appropriate information at a moment's notice, often in a crisis situation, he said. Compounded by the ever-changing nature of medical knowledge and the modern pressure to see as many patients as possible each day in order to maximize insurance payments, the situation sets up doctors and patients for costly and dangerous failures."[1]

Humility, fallibility, and uncertainty are not generally valued or modeled by medical mentors. Medical students and residents are taught that they can master this thing called diagnosis, when in reality it is a nearly impossible task. No one can make an accurate diagnosis every time. In his commencement speech at the Stanford University School of Medicine in June 2010, Dr. Atul Gawande told this group of new doctors:

> Half a century ago, medicine was neither costly nor effective. Since then, however, science has combated our ignorance. It has enumerated and identified, according to the international disease-classification system, more than 13,600 diagnoses—13,600 different ways our bodies can fail. And for each one we've discovered beneficial remedies—remedies that can reduce suffering, extend lives, and sometimes stop a disease altogether. But those remedies now include more than six thousand drugs and four thousand medical and surgical procedures. Our job in medicine is to make sure that all of this capability is deployed, town by town, in the right way at the right time, without harm or waste of resources, for every person alive. And we're struggling. There is no industry in the world with 13,600 different service lines to deliver.
>
> It should be no wonder that you have not mastered the understanding of them all. No one ever will.[2]

Because medical school and residency training promote the idea that doctors must come up with the correct diagnosis based on their own memories, physicians are destined to miss many diagnoses. Lawrence Weed, MD, who has spent a lifetime studying these issues, has said, "The physicians' unaided minds are incapable of recalling all the necessary knowledge from the literature and processing it with data from the unique patient. An epidemic of errors and waste is occurring as we persist in trying to do the impossible."[3] Dr. Weed and others who have recognized this problem suggest that physicians need to harness the power of information technology to avoid the high rate of missed or delayed diagnoses.

• **Number one: Overconfidence.** Mark Twain is reported to have said: "It ain't what you don't know that gets you into trouble. It's what you know for sure that just ain't so." Based on an analysis of available data, it is pretty clear that physician overconfidence is a major factor contributing to diagnostic disasters.[4] In their landmark study, "Overconfidence as a Cause of Diagnostic Error in Medicine," Drs. Berner and Graber suggest that overconfidence results from an attitude that might best be described as arrogance.[5]

Not Me!

Humans are frequently too confident about their own abilities to do complicated tasks without error. People complain about idiots on the highways but they overestimate their own driving skills all the time. Doctors are not immune to this tendency.

"Although clinicians are aware of the possibility for diagnostic error and that they are personally at risk, they believe that their own diagnoses are correct. Errors are made by someone else."[6]

Drs. Berner and Graber, *American Journal of Medicine*, May 2008

The problem with overconfidence is that doctors may not take the time or be willing to consider alternative possibilities for a patient's symptoms. One reason for the epidemic of overconfidence is that doctors rarely get feedback about diagnostic screwups. The doctor who makes a diagnosis on an outpatient usually doesn't hear when the diagnosis in the hospital is quite different. Either she is out of the loop, or else her colleagues may feel uncomfortable telling her that she messed up.[7] Without any way to check the accuracy of a diagnosis, a doctor can be both totally convinced of its appropriateness and totally wrong. In fact, doctors who were "completely certain" of their diagnosis before a patient died turned out in one study of autopsy results to be wrong 40 percent of the time.[8] Equally alarming, some studies have shown that the least competent clinicians are often the most confident.[9-11]

When a physician is overconfident about his diagnosis, he is less likely to be open to discussion with a patient. Any questioning may result in irritation or outright hostility. Such reactions interfere with communication and patient-provider partnerships. And when other members of the health care team, a nurse or a junior physician, sense something is wrong and challenge a more senior doctor, there is a likelihood that they will either be criticized or ignored. As a result, they often remain silent even in the face of a serious error.[12] This behavior reinforces the sin of overconfidence.

• **Number two: Information overload.** If you've ever had to clear away a stack of magazines you've been meaning to get to, but just couldn't keep up with, you may have an inkling of what your doctor faces. There are thousands of medical journals spewing out the latest research in a never-ending tidal wave. A busy clinician who comes home exhausted cannot possibly read all the medical journals in her area of expertise. Throw in the *Journal of the American Medical Association*, the *New England Journal of Medicine,* and several other general medical publications, and there is just no way to keep up. Even if your doctor could read half of the relevant research in his field, remembering it, especially at just the right moment to help with a difficult diagnosis, is impossible.

Let's take something as seemingly simple as a sore throat. What is the likelihood that an overworked family practice physician, an emergency department doctor, or a pediatrician will read an apparently abstruse article in the *Annals of Internal Medicine* titled "Expand the Pharyngitis Paradigm for Adolescents and Young Adults"?[13] But this article is a game changer that could save lives if doctors read and remembered it.

Most medical students and residents are taught that a bad sore throat should be cultured to see if it is caused by strep bacteria. If the test comes back positive, then the infection is treated with an appropriate antibiotic. The reason is that an untreated group A strep infection occasionally leads to rheumatic fever, which can be quite serious. If the test comes back negative, most physicians assume that the sore throat is not caused by anything serious, and that tincture of time is all that is necessary.

The article in the December 1, 2009, issue of the *Annals* reveals that this old way of thinking about sore throats is not good enough. Researchers have discovered that another bacterial infection called *Fusobacterium necrophorum* (dubbed F-throat by pediatrician Alan Greene) is at least as common among teenagers and young adults as strep. It doesn't show up on a rapid throat culture, and it can cause life-threatening complications.

Lisa Sanders, MD, writes the "Diagnosis" column for the *New York Times Magazine* and consults for the TV show *House.* In one column, she described a heartbreaking situation in which the diagnosis of F-throat was made too late.[14] The seventeen-year-old boy in her story had come down with a fever and sore throat, and his mother took him to see their family doctor the next day. Working on the horse-not-zebra principle, the family doctor diagnosed a strep throat and prescribed azithromycin (Zithromax, Zmax), a common antibiotic for strep throat. He didn't culture the boy's throat because it didn't seem necessary.

Instead of recovering quickly with antibiotic treatment, however, the young man continued to run a fever with shaking chills, and his sore throat got worse, localizing on one side of the neck. Although his parents took him to the hospital, the emergency department docs didn't think to look for F-throat, either. The antibiotics he was prescribed for presumed pneumonia were not effective against *Fusobacterium,* and by the time the doctors figured out what was making this boy so sick, it was too late to save his life.

His family doctor was devastated when he learned of this. Now, he cultures for F-throat as well as strep when a patient shows up with a sore throat. As he acknowledges, that might be overkill, but it also might save another person's life.

The current conventional wisdom is that F-throat primarily afflicts people between their early teens and early adult years, between the ages of fifteen and thirty. In that age group, it is just as common as strep. But even people outside that age range can suffer F-throat. Dr. Sanders has described one case of a forty-four-year-old mother who got the right diagnosis and treatment because her puzzled ear, nose, and throat specialist mentioned her case to a colleague who specialized in infectious disease. This expert recognized the possibility of F-throat from the brief description and recommended the antibiotic that saved her life.[15]

What's That Sore Throat?

Diagnosing F-throat is not a slam dunk. There is currently no rapid throat culture test for F-throat as there is for strep. As a result, doctors have to consider *Fusobacterium necrophorum* could be making a patient sick. Here are some clues:

• Bad sore throat

• Fever

• Pus in the back of the throat

• Swollen glands in the neck

• No cough

• Sore throat that does not get better in three to five days

• Swelling in the neck, especially on one side

• Night sweats and shivering

> Such symptoms require prompt treatment with the *right* antibiotic. Ask your doctor if you might have *Fusobacterium necrophorum*. Penicillin is the drug of choice. Cephalosporins such as cephalexin (Keflex), cefadroxil (Duricef), or cefaclor (Ceclor) also work. Macrolide antibiotics (azithromycin [Zithromax], clarithromycin [Biaxin], etc.) are ineffective.

Distinguishing F-throat from strep throat is just one small example of the huge amount of information that doctors need to master to make the right diagnosis. There's too much for any one person to remember, but, unfortunately, doctors don't always realize they should seek other resources. Using the Internet or computer-based decision support can be extremely helpful if a patient's symptoms are unusual. Drs. Newman-Toker and Pronovost cite the following: "For example, in a clinical scenario in which a patient describes rare symptoms, such as noting, 'I hear my eyes move,' the clinician may assume a mental illness, whereas an Internet search might identify a rare but treatable disorder such as superior canal dehiscence syndrome." This is an unusual condition of the middle ear that may affect balance and hearing.[16]

Half of Your Knowledge Is Wrong

As overwhelming as information overload is for a busy physician, changing information can be equally intimidating. Deans of medical schools are fond of quoting a message delivered decades ago to graduating students.

"Still we should keep in mind the words of a former leader of HMS [Harvard Medical School], Dr. C. Sidney Burwell, who was dean from 1935 to '49. At an HMS graduation in the late 1940s, he said '... Half of what we have taught you is wrong. Unfortunately, we don't know which half.' Though this quip may cause us to laugh, it is surely still true today."

Dean Jeffrey Flier, keynote address at the 2008 graduation ceremony of the Harvard Medical School

• **Number three: Going it alone.** We once got caught in a riptide off Ocracoke Island on the North Carolina's Outer Banks. A powerful current kept carrying us out to sea no matter how hard we tried to swim back toward shore. At some point we realized we were losing the battle and yelled for help. Fortunately, two brave souls heard our cries and came to our rescue with their floats. When we finally dragged our exhausted bodies onto the beach, we knew we had only survived thanks to the help of others.

Asking for help doesn't come easily to many physicians. To get into medical school you have to be a superb student and very competitive. One doctor described such people as "top guns." They are smart, bold, and driven. They are not necessarily people who instinctively know how to work well with others. Medical school and residency training don't usually teach teamwork or ego-free collaborative problem solving.[17] When faced with a diagnostic dilemma, such people are likely to try to solve the puzzle themselves. The trouble with this approach, however, is that if they get in over their heads, the patient may drown.

There are a number of resources that have evolved over the last few decades to aid physicians in both diagnostic and treatment decisions. One of the most powerful is something called a "knowledge coupler." This computer software enables patients to enter their symptoms and personal information into a computer. Then an enormous database assists the physician and patient to more accurately reach a diagnosis. There are other decision support systems available that enable physicians to tap the power of computers and the Internet rather than their faulty memories. Instead of embracing such technology, however, most physicians have resisted using these tools in the practice of medicine.[18-22]

Seeing Is Believing

Medical students and residents get relatively little dermatology training. As a result, diagnosing skin problems can sometimes be challenging for primary care physicians. Unusual skin conditions or atypical presentations of common problems can be hard to identify. That is why a picture is worth a thousand words.

A visual diagnostic decision support system (www.VisualDx.com) provides physicians an amazing opportunity to see a variety of skin problems in an intuitive way that can help identify what the problem might be. This powerful tool should be provided by every hospital and health care system in the country so that physicians would be encouraged to use it regularly for dermatologic diagnostic decisions. Patients can access a user-friendly version at www.skinsight.com.

Doctors, like baseball umpires, prefer to rely on their imperfect senses rather than modern technology to help in their decision making. Radiologists depend on their visual acuity and cognitive skills to analyze mammograms. But like umps, they make mistakes. Radiologists have resisted assessment tools designed to improve their accuracy in analyzing mammograms.[23]

When an umpire screws up, it is disappointing. For example, on June 2, 2010, Armando Galarraga pitched a perfect game (twenty-seven batters up, twenty-seven batters down), but a bad call by the first-base umpire cost Galarraga his place in history. When a radiologist screws up, it could delay a diagnosis of cancer and reduce the odds of a cure.

The same kind of bad decisions that occur in baseball used to be common in tennis. Umpires relied on their faulty eyesight to call balls in or out. Nowadays, sophisticated computer-assisted video replay tells instantly whether the ball was inside or outside the line. Shouldn't physicians use modern technology to improve their diagnostic decisions?

• **Number four: Tunnel vision.** In *How Doctors Think,* Dr. Jerome Groopman talks about something called anchoring: "a shortcut in thinking where a person doesn't consider multiple possibilities but quickly and firmly latches on to a single one, sure that he has thrown his anchor down just where he needs to be. You look at your map but your mind plays tricks on you—confirmation bias—because you see only the landmarks you expect to see and neglect those that should tell you that in fact you're still at sea. Your skewed reading of the map 'confirms' your mistaken assumption that you have reached your destination."[24]

Dr. Groopman describes the case of Blanche Begaye, a sixty-year-old Navajo woman who arrived at the emergency room (ER) complaining of trouble breathing. Initially, Blanche thought she had a nasty cold, for which she had taken "a few aspirin" and had drunk lots of orange juice. By the time she got to the ER, she was feeling awful, with a low-grade fever and rapid respiration.

The physician who examined her diagnosed "subclinical viral pneumonia," even though her breathing sounded okay, her chest X-ray was normal, and her blood test showed no white cell elevation typical of such an infection. An electrolyte test of her blood suggested acidity. There was no clear reason to assume pneumonia, but because this physician had seen dozens of other patients with viral pneumonia in the days preceding Blanche's visit to the ER, it was a quick and easy leap to that diagnosis.

The only problem was that the diagnosis was flat wrong. Blanche had overdosed on aspirin, which led to the electrolyte imbalance and rapid breathing. The incorrect diagnosis occurred because the doctor had anchored what seemed like the most obvious answer, even though there was conflicting evidence to suggest that something else was causing Blanche's symptoms. Fortunately, a more experienced doctor caught the mistake before it could cause irreparable harm.

Whether you call this kind of thinking process anchoring, tunnel vision, premature closure, or jumping to conclusions, it can be devastating to patients. Sadly, this is a common contributor to diagnostic screwups.

• **Number five: Time pressure.** One of the reasons that so many doctors end up jumping to conclusions is a lack of time to stop and think clearly. They're in a hurry all day long, dashing from one patient to the next. Visit just about any emergency department in the country, and you will see physicians and nurses trying to cope with an impossible workload. This can lead to brusque, even rude behavior. Dr. Jack Coulehan reported such an incident to his colleagues: "I saw a prime example of genuine arrogance in the hospital last week. A Spanish translator was devastated when a physician pushed her aside as he entered a non-English-speaking patient's room. 'I don't have time to spend talking,' he growled. 'I need to do this procedure right now.' And he did, while the frightened patient, who had presumably signed a consent form, had no idea what was happening. Unfortunately, such obnoxious behavior is not rare."[25]

Cutbacks in payments from insurance companies and the federal government have led many clinics and hospitals to encourage physicians to see more patients in less time. Some doctors have called this trend "hamster treadmill medicine" or "assembly-line medicine." Is it any wonder that physicians feel compelled to interrupt patients within twelve to twenty seconds after they start talking?

Dr. Peter Salgo is an internist and anesthesiologist at the Columbia University College of Physicians and Surgeons. His op-ed piece in the *New York Times* titled "The Doctor Will See You for Exactly Seven Minutes" is an indictment of the current way of practicing medicine: "The problem has been sneaking up on us for almost two decades. As health-care dollars became scarce in the 1980's and 90's, hospitals asked their business people to attend clinical meetings. The object was to see what doctors were doing that cost a lot of money, then to try and do things more efficiently.... Publicly traded H.M.O.'s, for example, began restricting doctors to an average seven-minute 'encounter' with each customer. This apparently kept shareholders happy. But it reduced the doctor-patient relationship to a financial concept in a business school term paper."[26]

The problem with time pressure is that it increases the risk of diagnostic errors. Without an adequate amount of time to listen attentively to a patient tell her whole story, including seemingly irrelevant details, a busy clinician may miss something important. To discern what is really causing the patient distress, a physician needs time to consider a variety of possibilities and then think things through clearly. Just as we can't put a complicated jigsaw puzzle together in seven minutes, a clinician can't diagnose confusing symptoms in seven minutes. She shouldn't have to try.

• **Number six: Missing test results.** When we were graduate students at the University of Michigan in Ann Arbor, we relied on the student health service. Terry was regularly falling asleep after eating fruit yogurt and an apple for lunch, and a physician ordered a glucose tolerance test for her. He suspected she might be suffering from reactive hypoglycemia, a condition in which blood sugar levels zoom up quickly after eating a high-carb meal and then drop dramatically. In this test the person drinks an intensely sugary drink quickly, and then over the next few hours blood is drawn periodically, and glucose levels are monitored carefully. This test can diagnose diabetes as well as hypoglycemia.

Since we never heard a word about the test results, we assumed everything was fine. Terry continued to eat high-carbohydrate lunches and continued to get drowsy in the afternoon. Several months later she had to go to student health because of a dermatology concern. The physician who saw her glanced at the top paper in her medical chart and casually mentioned, "Oh, I see you have reactive hypoglycemia." Terry was flabbergasted. He showed her the chart and how her blood glucose levels dropped dramatically after the high-sugar drink. His advice was to eat several small high-protein snacks throughout the day. That simple advice made a huge difference for Terry. If he had not told Terry about the lab results, she would not have known she needed to change her eating habits. Whether her high-carbohydrate diet would have put her at risk of type 2 diabetes remains controversial.

Missing Lab Results

"Ordering and following up on outpatient laboratory and imaging tests consumes large amounts of physician time and is important in the diagnostic process. Diagnostic errors are the most frequent cause of malpractice claims in the United States; testing-related mistakes can lead to serious diagnostic errors. There are many steps in the testing process, which extends from ordering a test to providing appropriate follow-up; an error in any one of these steps can have lethal consequences."

Lawrence P. Casalino, MD, et al.,

in *Archives of Internal Medicine*, June 22, 2009[27]

You might think our story was an isolated example about a student health service that may have been a bit disorganized. We assure you that this kind of screwup is not unusual today in almost any hospital or medical practice in the country. A study published in the *Archives of Internal Medicine* disclosed that one out of fourteen patients with abnormal test results never heard about them from their doctors. Such stats are scary, but it gets worse. In some practices, as many as one-quarter of the patients were not notified of their anomalous results when they should have been.[28] The authors concluded that such failures to inform are common.

Missing PSA Results

Phil (not his real name) was extremely conscientious about having his prostate tested because his father had developed prostate cancer. Phil went to one of the leading cancer centers for oversight. His internist was supposed to send his PSA (prostate-specific antigen) test results to the specialists to track potential problems. Since Phil never heard about problems, he assumed all was well. It wasn't!

None of his PSA test results were sent to the cancer center for evaluation. Eventually, however, his PSA became quite elevated, and he was diagnosed with prostate cancer. His PSA levels had been rising, but Phil had not been informed of the situation. If his doctor's office had been better organized for sharing test results, his prostate cancer could have been treated at a much earlier stage.

What these statistics mean is that an extraordinary number of people never learn about abnormal results from a pathology report or a blood test or even a CT (computerized tomography) scan. Part of the reason for this kind of screwup is that many medical practices are disorganized and have not implemented procedures to monitor and transmit patient data. Management of test results is not something that is taught in medical school. Some doctors happen to do it really well, while others routinely drop the ball. Never assume no news is good news. It could just be that your lab results got buried on your doctor's desk and were eventually filed away without anyone paying attention to a potential problem.

• **Number seven: Ignoring drug side effects.** Just about every drug known to man has the potential to cause some side effects in some people. So how does a doctor who wants to do the best for his patient justify prescribing a medicine that could cause heart attacks, strokes, life-threatening liver failure, or kidney disease, to name just a few drug-induced side effects?

To cope with what has to be incredible cognitive dissonance, many physicians respond to the idea of drug side effects by, first, minimizing their likelihood and, second, denying their very existence. Take statins, for example. Few medications have captivated physicians more than statins. Experts estimate that in any given year anywhere from 11 million to 30 million people take a medication like rosuvastatin (Crestor), atorvastatin (Lipitor), lovastatin (Mevacor), pravastatin (Pravachol), or simvastatin (Zocor). Since these cholesterol-lowering drugs were launched over two decades ago, they have brought in over $250 billion for the pharmaceutical industry.[29]

Many doctors believe that statins are magic bullets against heart disease. Some insist that any patient with a slightly elevated cholesterol level should take a statin or risk hellfire and damnation or, at the very least, death. Statins do reduce the risk of heart attacks and strokes for people with clearly identified heart disease. They do *not*, however, seem to prolong life in otherwise healthy folks who are taking statins to prevent problems in the first place. An analysis of eleven clinical trials involving over 65,000 people produced no evidence that statins saved lives in this population, even though they had risk factors such as elevated cholesterol levels.[30]

Following the "first, do no harm" mantra, one would think that physicians would be especially careful about prescribing statins for healthy people and be vigilant about side effects, but that is often not the case. We have received hundreds of messages from people who have experienced a range of severe side effects from statins. Many have been chastised for stopping their medication, and doctors often denied that the patients' problems were related to the drug.

Statin Complaints

"I am sixty years old, and in excellent overall health with no history of heart disease. Because my cholesterol was high on one blood test, my doctor immediately put me on Lipitor. I wanted to try diet and exercise first, but she negated that idea.

"Over the course of two years on Lipitor, I developed terrible pains in my wrists, thumbs, feet, and legs. Then my eyebrows, eyelashes, and head hair began to fall out. I also got increasingly 'spacey' and started forgetting words and names. My doctor refused to accept that Lipitor could cause any of this.

"This may sound arrogant, but I simply quit taking it. My hair and eyelashes have grown back, and *all* muscle and joint pain is gone. My memory is also back to normal."

Susan, August 7, 2009

The reports we have received mirror the results of a survey conducted by researchers at the University of California at San Diego.[31-32] This survey of 650 patients experiencing side effects on statins found that the majority of these patients discussed the side effects with their physicians, nearly always at the patient's instigation. Physicians rarely asked about such side effects. Patients reported that their doctors were far more likely to deny any connection between the drug and the problem than to affirm a possible connection. This was true even for reactions that have been well documented in the medical literature, such as muscle pain,[33] which can affect as many as 10 to 15 percent of people taking statins.[34-35] Other less well-known but documented reactions covered in the survey included nerve problems (neuropathy)[36] and cognitive difficulties.[37-38]

When doctors fail to take patient accounts of side effects seriously, they are not likely to report the problems, either to the Food and Drug Administration or as a case report in the medical literature.[39] As a result, other physicians also have more trouble making a connection. That can slow the recognition of seemingly unrelated side effects such as cataracts (which have been linked to statins in a surprisingly high proportion of patients).[40] Refusing to consider a possible connection between the patient's symptoms and the drug also interferes with the ability to address the problem the patient is experiencing and correct it.

Medication Merry-Go-Round

"First I was put on Zocor to control my cholesterol. That caused restless leg syndrome (RLS), so I was prescribed Requip. I then became depressed and was prescribed the antidepressant Lexapro. It made me into a zombie, so I was prescribed a low dose of Ritalin, a stimulant drug for ADHD [attention deficit/hyperactivity disorder].

"I developed a mild heart arrhythmia [likely an effect of the Ritalin] and was prescribed a calcium channel blocker (CCB) to control the heart rhythm. I took the CCB for about three weeks and felt so bad I wanted to commit suicide.

"When I tried to refill the Zocor at the local pharmacy instead of through mail order, the pharmacist told me he could not give me the CCB and a statin at the same time. That did it for me. I had been a zombie for far too long.

"I swore off all prescription medicine. Without all these pills, my mental fog lifted, the terrible muscle spasms I had everywhere relaxed, and I no longer had RLS."

K. Y., October 23, 2007

We don't condone people stopping their prescription drugs without their doctors' involvement and advice. But we hate it when doctors just prescribe more medicine to treat drug side effects, instead of stepping back to see if there is some other way to accomplish the goal. Every problem this person developed was a medication side effect—and each one was treated with yet another drug that caused an additional complication.

• **Number eight: Follow-up failure.** One of the reasons that doctors sometimes don't realize how frequently their diagnoses miss the mark is that they rarely get feedback on how the story ends.[41] Under normal circumstances, the emergency department doctor won't hear back from the physicians upstairs in the hospital. The specialist and the primary care physician may communicate, but perhaps not as much as one might hope. The patient with a puzzling constellation of symptoms may get passed from one doctor to another to a third or even a fourth before a diagnosis can be reached. At that point, the patient is generally so relieved to finally understand what is going on that she may not inform all the doctors she saw along this torturous path.

Major league pitchers get constant feedback from their coaches. So do quarterbacks. In fact, no professional athlete can improve without constructive criticism from experts who analyze every aspect of his game. And yet most physicians get little if any feedback about their diagnostic bloopers. Without this kind of follow-up, it is very difficult to (1) be aware of diagnostic errors and (2) improve their strategy in the future. Our fragmented health care system makes this a challenge.

• **Number nine: Hurried hand-offs.** This is a biggie! Transitions are an Achilles' heel of medicine, whether in a hospital or going from one doctor to another. Think airplanes for a moment. When a plane takes off, it is monitored by the air traffic control tower of the departure airport. But once the plane leaves the range of that tower, it is handed off to the next control area in a very organized fashion. This way, there is constant monitoring so that there are no collisions or other mishaps.

When patients go from one doctor to another, there is no organized system for hand-offs. This is often true even within the same hospital. Many diagnostic mistakes take place in the emergency department (ED). If you have ever had to go to the emergency room, you know what a bizarre setting it has become. There is almost always a waiting room full of people, and the wait time is interminable. Unless you are bleeding on the floor or having a heart attack or a stroke, you could easily be there for many hours before you are seen. The people who work in the ED are harried and often have to make snap decisions under pressure. In one study of malpractice claims, "approximately half of the missed diagnoses (52 percent) involved emergency physicians."[42]

Hand-off Catastrophe

A man went to the emergency department (ED) of his local hospital complaining of lower back pain. He mentioned to a nurse that he was also having bladder problems and some numbness in his legs, but when the doctor came bustling into the room, he asked what the problem was and the patient focused primarily on his back pain.

During the hand-off between the nurse and the doctor, the information about the bladder problems and numbness fell through a crack and was not communicated. Because this was not the first time the patient had ended up in the ED with a back problem, the doctor was not overly concerned. As a result, the patient was released from the emergency room with a diagnosis of a back problem.

Several hours later, he was admitted to another hospital, where he was diagnosed with cauda equina syndrome (CES). This is a condition caused by compression of nerves in the lower spinal cord. It causes symptoms such as back pain and urinary retention and then incontinence, leg pain, and weakness. CES usually requires emergency surgery. Left untreated, it can lead to paralysis of the legs as well as permanent loss of bowel and bladder control. That is what happened to this patient.

When the patient needs blood work, an X-ray, and a CT (computerized tomography) or an MRI (magnetic resonance imaging) scan, it can take hours for the results to get back to the doctor who ordered them. If a shift change occurred in the meantime and that doctor has gone home, the replacement physician may not connect all the dots in a timely fashion.[43] Transitions are trouble, so make sure the providers are paying extra-careful attention during any hand-off.

• **Number ten: Communication breakdown.** Whether during a hand-off or at some other time, communication failures cause problems. When patients don't get to tell their whole story, important clues are missed. When doctors don't communicate all relevant details to colleagues, the diagnosis and treatment can go horribly wrong.

Disastrous Miscommunication

A fifty-year-old man went to the emergency department with chest pain. The doctors thought he might be having a heart attack, so they admitted him and put him on an anticoagulant. It turned out that his chest pain was actually caused by an inflamed gallbladder.

But although the correct diagnosis was eventually made and the patient was scheduled for gallbladder surgery, no one changed the orders for the intravenous anticoagulant. He continued to receive it right up to the time of his surgery the following day and even got another dose after the surgery. Neither the surgeon nor the anesthesiologist realized that the man was receiving an anticoagulant, which is contraindicated for surgery because it increases the risk of excessive bleeding.

Later that evening, the man's blood pressure dropped, and he had trouble breathing. He had been bleeding into his abdomen. Even though the surgeon operated on him again to remove all the fluid and then put him in intensive care, he did not survive. In this case, the communication failure did not prevent the correct diagnosis, but it put the patient at mortal risk.[44]

Patients sometimes complain about having to repeat their whole history and all their symptoms to each health care provider they see, but instead of feeling miffed, they should take advantage of the opportunity. The medical student who seems so attentive may never speak to the nurse on duty. The nurse, who has written a detailed account in the chart, may not speak with the resident who does rounds. The attending physician may be so busy that she never looks at the chart or talks to the nurse or the resident. As a result, assuming that telling a story once is enough could be a major mistake.

An analysis of malpractice claims shows that communication failures contribute to other sources of misdiagnosis. They include an incomplete medical history, missing medical tests, or inadequate follow-up on tests.[45]

These are just our top 10 reasons why doctors screw up diagnoses. There may be others, but there are things that doctors and patients can do to reduce diagnostic errors. In the next chapter, we offer some tips on preventing these serious screwups.

CHAPTER 5

PREVENTING DIAGNOSTIC PROBLEMS

Humans are incredibly adaptable. You can put us into the most bizarre situations, and we somehow learn to cope; eventually, we even begin to accept an untenable situation as almost normal. Unfortunately, this happens in medicine, too. Arrogance, ego, and hierarchy have become entrenched within the culture of medicine. This has led to what Dr. Peter Pronovost describes as "normalization of deviance." It prevents a nurse who sees a physician making a potentially deadly mistake from speaking up, either because she fears being ignored or "having her head bitten off."[1]

Arrogance vs. Humility

"Perhaps the most difficult virtue to understand and practice is humility, which seems out of place in a medical culture characterized by arrogance, assertiveness, and a sense of entitlement. Countercultural though it is, humility need not suggest weakness or lack of self-confidence. On the contrary, humility requires toughness and emotional resilience. Humility in medicine manifests itself as unflinching self-awareness, empathic openness to others, and a deep appreciation of and gratitude for the privilege of caring for sick persons."[2]

Jack Coulehan, MD, MPH, in *Annals of Internal Medicine*, August 3, 2010

For decades, hospital administrators and chief medical officers have accepted infections in hospitals as normal, just as their predecessors did in the nineteenth century. When Hungarian physician Ignaz Semmelweis demonstrated in 1847 that puerperal fever ["childbed fever"] could be dramatically reduced if obstetricians disinfected their hands before delivering a baby, he was ignored, ridiculed, and harassed by his peers.

In fact, Dr. Semmelweis was committed to an insane asylum, where he died. We hope our modern-day crusaders for patient safety fare better.

Dr. Pronovost and his colleagues have demonstrated that if doctors and nurses followed a five-point checklist, they could dramatically reduce catheter-related bloodstream infections in intensive care units.[3] Such infections cause a great deal of suffering and many deaths. To minimize them, health care providers had to put aside their egos and their hierarchies and work together as a team for the benefit of patients. We think diagnostic errors could also be diminished if health care providers, patients, and families all worked together as a team. The new term for this approach is *participatory medicine.*

Participatory Medicine

"Participatory Medicine is a movement in which networked patients shift from being mere passengers to responsible drivers of their health, and in which providers encourage and value them as full partners."[4]

To have an impact on the millions of misdiagnoses that occur each year physicians are going to have to overcome some ingrained behaviors. Changing an entrenched medical culture will be incredibly challenging. Medical schools will have to select students for their creativity, empathy, and problem-solving ability as well as their memorization skills. We need more team players than "top guns." Arrogance and overconfidence have to go. While it is probably unrealistic to expect humility and vulnerability from most health care professionals, we do need them to accept that fallibility is a component of the human condition. It is probably asking too much of physicians to embrace uncertainty, since their training conditions them to shun this concept. Nevertheless, uncertainty is a reality in medicine. Although some signs and symptoms are obvious indicators of a particular condition, many others are ambiguous and require sleuthing, intuition, testing, and modern technology to determine a correct diagnosis.

Accepting Uncertainty

"In medicine, humility feels like a square peg in a round hole. Toughness, confidence, and assertiveness—yes. Drama, angst, and celebrity—yes. But prudence and humility—no, not exactly. We revere the concept of compassionate care but are skeptical about seeming to be weak; wishy-washy; or even deceptive, as in 'false modesty.' Patients, too, may question the competence of physicians who too readily acknowledge their limitations."[5]

Jack Coulehan, MD, MPH, in *Annals of Internal Medicine*, August 3, 2010

Ultimately, the most important component to successful diagnosis will be good communication and collaboration between patients, nurses, and physicians. That requires attentive listening by health professionals. Patients need to be able to tell their stories without being interrupted. Seemingly trivial details may provide the key to unlocking a mystery.

When Something Is Just Not Right

Dr. David Newman-Toker (N-T) is a neurologist at Johns Hopkins. A patient, who happened to be a nurse, was referred to him by another physician. The woman believed her symptoms (dizziness and double vision) were brought on by a medication she was taking.

Dr. N-T was concerned enough that he encouraged her to go an emergency department so she could be checked out for a transient ischemic attack (TIA), or a pre-stroke. According to Dr. N-T:

"She was examined quickly, found to have no persistent abnormalities on her examination and to have a normal CT [computerized tomography] scan of the brain and was told to go home.

"It was only through an added layer of insistence on my part that we were able to convince her to go to another hospital, where we admitted her and found out that this was indeed a transient ischemic attack in the brain and that she was at significant risk for stroke. We gave her an appropriate treatment to prevent that and she did well."

The red flag that tipped off Dr. N-T was the fact that the patient had taken her medicine the prior evening, and when she woke that morning, there were no symptoms. They came on around 11:00 A.M., lasted for 30 or 40 minutes, went away, and then returned around 1:00 P.M. for another 20 minutes. The medication hypothesis seemed implausible to him.[6] That nagging doubt turned out to be right.

Top 10 Questions to Ask to Reduce Diagnostic Disasters

1. What are my primary concerns and symptoms?
2. How confident are you about this diagnosis?
3. What further tests might be helpful to improve your confidence?
4. Will the test(s) you are proposing change the treatment plan in any way?
5. Are there any findings or symptoms that don't fit your diagnosis or that contradict it?
6. What else could it be?
7. Can you facilitate a second opinion by providing me my medical records?
8. When should I expect to see my test results? Will you call with them, or will they come by mail or electronically?
9. What resources can you recommend for me to learn more about my diagnosis?
10. May I contact you by e-mail if my symptoms change or if I have an important question? If so, what is your e-mail address?

• **Number one: What are my primary concerns and symptoms?**
Think about a conversation with your physician as if it were a noisy cell

phone conversation with a friend. If that person goes into a cell-phone dead zone, there can be critical dropouts. Your doctor may be preoccupied or just not hearing everything you are saying clearly. When pilots and air traffic controllers speak to each other, they have a carefully choreographed system to verify that each has heard the other correctly. The same thing is essential when you tell your story to your physician. Ask her to "teach back" to you what she heard. That way you will be sure she got all the key points.

• **Number two: How confident are you about this diagnosis?** Some diagnoses are obvious. You went walking in the woods, and the next day you have itchy red bumps on your skin. Those three-pointed leaves you touched climbing over that big log were indeed poison ivy. Dizziness, on the other hand, can be triggered by all sorts of things, from medication to a neurological condition. As Dr. David Newman-Toker pointed out, getting the diagnosis right requires a healthy degree of open-mindedness and the realization that something else might be going on. Encourage your doctor to share his level of uncertainty about your diagnosis.

• **Number three: What further tests might improve your level of confidence?** This is a slippery slope. On the one hand, you want an accurate diagnosis. On the other, you do not want to undergo expensive, risky procedures that may not provide much useful information. CT scans can be very helpful in diagnosing certain puzzling symptoms; they can, for example, assist in verifying acute appendicitis. They can also be abused. A routine abdominal CT scan exposes a patient to roughly the equivalent of 400 X-rays. That is a *lot* of radiation. A study in the *Archives of Internal Medicine* suggests that the radiation from CT scans done in 2007 alone will eventually result in 29,000 cancers and 15,000 deaths.[7] Finding the balance between accuracy, affordability, and safety is critical to any decision to seek additional testing.

• **Number four: Will the test(s) you are proposing change the treatment plan in any way?** Most doctors are curious. That's a good thing. They want to know what is causing your symptoms. But sometimes their curiosity can lead to expensive, invasive tests that hurt and may not change anything about your treatment. An eighty-three-year-old man who complains that he has to get up frequently at night to pee almost assuredly has an enlarged prostate. If his doctor orders a blood test for PSA (prostate-specific antigen) and it is elevated, the doctor then might be tempted to order a prostate biopsy to check for cancer, which is painful and can lead to complications of its own, such as infection. Many experts now refrain from such testing because even if cancer were detected, they would generally discourage aggressive treatment in an older man, since the side effects of the treatment may outweigh the benefits.[8]

• **Number five: Are there any findings or symptoms that don't fit your diagnosis or that contradict it?** Once a doctor anchors onto a diagnosis, it can be hard for him to dismiss it, even if there is evidence that doesn't quite fit the pattern. In her book *Every Patient Tells a Story: Medical Mysteries and the Art of Diagnosis*, Lisa Sanders, MD, describes the puzzling case of Graciela. She woke one day feeling as if her legs were on fire. The pain continued, and her left leg became weak. She developed a dry, irritating cough and became short of breath after the slightest exertion. A chest X-ray showed some cloudy patches in the lung.

After undergoing countless blood tests, CT (computerized tomography) and MRI (magnetic resonance imaging) scans of her head and spine, and a lung biopsy, the various specialists determined Graciela was probably suffering from scleroderma, an autoimmune disease involving connective tissue. A rheumatologist called in to confirm the diagnosis didn't buy it. For one thing, she didn't have thickening of the skin, a classic sign of scleroderma. Careful review of the lung biopsy revealed a granuloma and the real culprit, sarcoidosis, "a mysterious chronic disease characterized by inflammation of tissues that often display the unusual granuloma collection of cells."[9] Patients need to be informed when something doesn't quite fit with the diagnosis. You may have to ask, though, because this kind of information may not be readily volunteered.

• **Number six: What else could it be?** This is huge! If we had time to ask our doctor only one question, this is probably the Big Kahuna. *Always* ask this question regardless of how sure your physician is that he has your diagnosis nailed. As we have pointed out earlier, the more confident the doctor, the greater the likelihood of a diagnostic error.

Dr. Sanders describes the case of David P. in her book. Over the course of a couple of months, he had made four trips to the emergency department complaining of chest pain, trouble breathing, and numbness in hands and fingers. Initially, the doctors thought he was having a heart attack, but all the tests turned out negative. Over time, David's fingers became so weak he could hardly hold things. He also complained of fatigue, constipation, and numbness in his feet. Finally, a doctor noticed that a prior blood test had revealed anemia, an unusual symptom in a twenty-seven-year-old 240-pound weight lifter. Although it had been ignored, this symptom was the key to unlocking the mystery. Another blood test revealed a severe vitamin B_{12} deficiency brought on by an autoimmune disorder called pernicious anemia. Low levels of this B vitamin could account for his symptoms. Vitamin B_{12} injections reversed the symptoms. Never forget to ask "What else could it be?"

• **Number seven: Can you facilitate a second opinion by providing me my medical records?** This is hard. Really hard! Even though patients have the legal right to review or obtain a copy of their medical records, it takes chutzpah to ask a doctor to provide a copy. Many people fear that they will antagonize their health care provider by requesting this document. Some doctors will be annoyed, but the growing movement toward electronic medical records is encouraging patient access. Many health systems are setting up patient "portals" through which patients can make appointments, pay bills, view lab results, and sometimes even see portions of the medical record online. If you request paper records, there is almost always a per page copying fee. Electronic records should be free. Ask for a copy of your medical records for your files. This way you can correct errors that may exist and keep track of your progress. Most important, you can share your record and test results with another physician should you seek a second or third opinion.

• **Number eight: When should I expect to see my test results? Will you call with them, or will they come by mail or electronically?** Doctors and doctors' offices can be disorganized, just like the rest of us. They are human, after all. The trouble is that their disorganization can have life-threatening ramifications. As mentioned previously in this book, a study of how well doctors notified patients about abnormal test results revealed that abnormal results were *not* reported to patients one out of fourteen times.[10] In some practices, though, unusual results were not transmitted to patients one out of *four* times. Since you have no way of knowing whether your doctor is organized or cavalier about communicating test results, you need to ask specifically about when you should expect to hear from his or her staff. If you don't hear from the doctor by that date, call the office and ask the receptionist or nurse to assist in accessing the information.

Missing Information

Joe had a funny-looking mole on his left shoulder blade. It bled easily and was a bit itchy. When the dermatologist looked at it, his comment was, "That mole looks a little strange."

The doctor removed it for biopsy. Over the next several days Joe convinced himself that the "strange" mole must be melanoma.

Days and then weeks went by with no word from the dermatologist. Eventually, Joe called the dermatologist's office. Days later, the call was returned. The pathology report had been buried under papers on the doctor's desk. Since everything was normal, the dermatologist didn't think this was a priority and promptly forgot about it.

Joe breathed a huge sigh of relief, but weeks of stress and anxiety could have been prevented by a reassuring phone call.

• **Number nine: What resources can you recommend for me to learn more about my diagnosis?** When a doctor gives you a scary diagnosis, it can be overwhelming. Even something fairly common like diabetes or hypertension can seem overwhelming. When you get home and process the information, you may be tempted to turn to Dr. Google for more insight about your condition.

We are all in favor of searching the Web for health information. Robert Greenwald, MD, wrote a letter to the *New England Journal of Medicine* describing a case at his hospital. An infant had diarrhea, an unusual rash ("alligator skin"), and a variety of immunological abnormalities. None of the attending physicians or house staff could decide what the correct diagnosis was. A junior physician diagnosed a rare condition called IPEX (immunodeficiency, polyendocrinopathy, enteropathy, X-linked). "How did you make that diagnosis?" asked the professor. She responded, "Well, I had the skin biopsy report, and I had a chart of the immunologic tests. So I entered the salient features into Google and it popped right up."[11]

The Web has an amazing amount of helpful information if used skillfully, but people may also end up scaring themselves to death with inaccurate diagnoses. Patients can benefit from this incredible tool if they are selective and consult their doctor for interpretations and recommendations. (For example, if someone has a skin problem, he can go to www.skinsight.com to get visual help on potential diagnoses.) Asking your doctor to point you in the right direction for reliable websites and information can help turn your physician into a partner.

• **Number ten: May I contact you by e-mail if my symptoms change or if I have an important question? If so, what is your e-mail address?** Be prepared for your doctor to say no. Most doctors reserve their e-mail for family, friends, and colleagues. Doctors seem to fear that they will be inundated by long messages and questions from patients that will take up significant amounts of their time.[12] They worry about the impersonal nature of e-mail, inappropriate use by patients during emergencies, increased liability, breached security, and lack of reimbursement for their time.[13]

Although there is not a lot of research on e-mail communication in medicine, the doctors' fears appear to be unfounded. One study noted that in a pediatric rheumatology practice, e-mail actually *reduced* the amount of time physicians spent answering questions as compared with using the telephone. Trying to reach a physician by phone is an incredibly frustrating experience for patients, since they often have to deal with a phone tree or leave a message with a receptionist. Then there is the likelihood of telephone tag, which is frustrating for everyone. The research also demonstrated that patients did not find e-mail impersonal; instead, they reported that it improved communication. Most telling of all, after the study was completed, the number of pediatricians in this practice who adopted e-mail access went from 25 percent to 80 percent.[14]

Patient-Physician E-mail Access

"Answering patient questions by e-mail was 57 percent faster than using the telephone for the physician. The physician received 1.2 e-mails per day from patients. The families who responded to the survey agreed that patient-physician e-mail increased access to the physician and improved the quality of care."[15]

The best argument for e-mail between patients and their physicians would be improved care. That is precisely what researchers at Kaiser Permanente found. They examined more than 500,000 secure e-mail strings between system doctors and patients between October 2007 and December 2008. Patients with diabetes scored better on measures of health quality if they communicated with their doctors by e-mail.[16] Patients were better able to let doctors know of changes in their condition, ask about lab results, and inquire about drug dosages. The doctors at Kaiser Permanente averaged between two and twelve messages in a workday, a reasonable number even for a busy physician.

E-mail Etiquette

If your physician is willing to give you her e-mail address, here are some guidelines:

- *Never* use e-mail in an emergency. Call 911 and go to your local emergency department!
- Keep your e-mail communications concise, formal, and relevant. Do not write paragraphs. They will overwhelm your physician.
- Your e-mail will likely become part of your medical record, so do not include anything that you are not willing to share with other members of the health care team or anyone else who has permission to view your records.
- Recognize that unless your physician has a password-protected Web-based portal with encryption security, your message may not be 100 percent secure. Of course, that is true for most e-mail sent to friends and family. Really private communications should be saved for telephone conversations or face-to-face meetings.

We think these questions are critical to making sure you get the right diagnosis. We also recognize that you are likely to have only a few minutes with your doctor, so it is unrealistic to tell your story completely and ask all ten questions. That's why it is essential to prioritize. Make sure you focus on the key problems you are experiencing. Doctors hate it when they put their hand on the door to leave the room and the patient says something like, "Oh doctor, there's one other thing I forgot to mention. I have been coughing up blood for the last six days." That is a game changer and should be the *first* thing you mention, not the last.

We have provided all ten of our questions on page 69 for you to photocopy and take to your next appointment. Determine in advance which five you think are most important for any given visit. Do not be adversarial. Ask these questions in a friendly, conversational man-ner. You want your physician to be your ally, not your enemy. From our vantage point, you should always make numbers 1, 6, and 8 part of the conversation, but every interaction is unique. That is why you should try to plan ahead.

CHAPTER 6

TOP 10 SCREWUPS DOCTORS MAKE WHEN PRESCRIBING

1. Failing to disclose drug side effects
2. Creating obstacles to reporting symptoms
3. Ignoring drug-induced symptoms
4. Overriding medication alerts
5. Being oblivious to drug prices
6. Not knowing actual drug effectiveness
7. Relying on surrogate markers
8. Not checking for drug interactions
9. Not staying up to date on new research
10. Not reporting drug problems to the FDA

Doctors prescribe an amazing number of drugs. At the time of this writing, roughly 4 billion prescriptions are dispensed each year.[1] If the average number of pills in a bottle is 30, that is at least 120 billion pills, or over 390 tablets and capsules for every man, woman, and child in the United States each year. By the way, the bill for all those pills is more than $300 billion. That does not take into account the number of medications dispensed in hospitals or nursing homes or all the over-the-counter medications that are consumed annually.

With so many people taking so many drugs, it should come as no surprise that there are a tremendous number of problems, known in doctorspeak as ADEs (adverse drug events). In truth, no one has a clue how many people suffer or die from serious drug-induced side effects each year and how many ADEs could have been prevented.[2] Researchers using a probability model have concluded that pharmaceuticals are responsible for more than 17 million visits to emergency rooms and 8.7 million hospitalizations each year.[3] They also predict that 300,000 people die each year from medicines that were supposed to help them.[4-5] The prestigious Institute of Medicine reviewed a variety of studies and concluded that "there are at least 1.5 million preventable ADEs that occur in the United States each year. The true number may be much higher."[6]

Some of the country's leading patient safety experts have discovered that "much, *much* higher" could be closer to the truth. They studied adverse drug events in primary care practices and concluded that "as many as 7.8 million ADEs could be prevented or ameliorated if patients and their physicians communicated better and if physicians acted more reliably to address medication symptoms."[7]

These numbers are so mind boggling that it's hard to comprehend their significance. These are medications that are supposed to relieve suffering, cure us when we are ill, and prevent catastrophic complications of chronic illness such as heart attacks and strokes. And yet millions are being harmed each year from medicine, making adverse drug events one of the leading causes of death in the United States.[8] This is the antithesis of the old admonition "Don't let the cure be worse than the disease."

• **Number one: Failure to disclose drug side effects.** Patient safety researchers discovered that physicians ignored drug-related symptoms one out of four times.[9] In other words, when patients complained that their medicine was causing side effects such as dizziness or difficulty with balance, headache, rash, insomnia, or muscle aches, doctors failed to address 26 percent of their "confirmed" symptoms.

Side Effect Denial

"I am frustrated with my doctor's lack of response to my side effect from the blood pressure drug diltiazem HCl ER. Since I have been on this drug, my sleep has been interrupted at least three times a night, as I have to get up to relieve myself. Faithfully, I have reported this to my cardiologist for the past three visits. He replies straight-facedly, 'This medicine does not have that side effect.' I quote to him from a nurses' drug book I used as a reference: '2 percent of patients may have polyuria, nocturia, or frequency of urination,' and apparently I am one of those two in a hundred."

Although we find these statistics on physicians' failure to disclose or address drug side effects shocking, we are not surprised. Over the last thirty-five years, we have received thousands of letters, e-mail messages, and posts to our website like the example in the preceding sidebar, suggesting that too many physicians fail to inform patients adequately about common or serious drug side effects. They may also ignore symptoms when a patient complains. One classic example (discussed on page 31) has to do with a class of blood pressure–lowering medications called ACE (angiotension-converting enzyme) inhibitors. These are drugs such as benazepril (Lotensin), captopril (Capoten), enalapril (Vasotec), fosinopril (Monopril), ramipril (Altace), and quinapril (Accupril). Over 130 million prescriptions are dispensed for these drugs each year.

One of the most common and disturbing side effects of ACE inhibitors is a cough that cannot be controlled by cough medicine. If a patient experiences this symptom, the only solution is to switch him to a different kind of blood pressure medicine. We have heard from an incredible number of patients that (1) they were never informed that their medicine could cause a cough and (2) when they started coughing violently (to the point of throwing up), the cause of their cough was not addressed.

Why in the world would a physician not mention such a side effect when writing a new prescription? And if someone complained of coughing, why wouldn't a different blood pressure medicine be substituted? Some experts have speculated that doctors "erroneously believe that giving patients information about the possible adverse effects of a medication will increase the possibility that the patients will experience symptoms. In fact, Ambulatory Quality Improvement Project investigators found that patients reported fewer problems with medications when they were told in advance about potential adverse effects."[10-11] In 1970, an editorial in the *Journal of the American Medical Association* (*JAMA*) made it crystal clear: "When a physician prescribes a drug, he has an obligation to warn the patient about the drug's potential for causing adverse reactions, especially the more serious ones."[12]

Informed consent is a concept understood by every surgeon in America. No procedure can be performed until a patient is told about the risks and benefits of what they are about to undergo. Patients even have to sign a form that confirms that they understood what was communicated and grant their permission to proceed. The same concept should hold true whenever a drug is prescribed. And yet, more than four decades after the *JAMA* editorial, many physicians still fail to warn patients about drug side effects in ways that can be remembered and acted upon.

What Happens When Patients Are Not Informed

We heard a tragic story from a mother whose twenty-six-year-old daughter was being treated for Graves' disease, an overactive thyroid gland. She was prescribed Tapazole (methimazole) to suppress her thyroid, but she was not told that this drug could reduce her ability to fight infection by reducing her production of white blood cells.

Despite a clear warning in the prescribing information to have patients report sore throat, fever, or other symptoms of infection, this young woman was treated for many sore throats, strep infections, tonsillitis, and gingivitis without a blood test. The doctor treating her failed to connect her series of infections with an adverse effect of her treatment for Graves' disease. When she finally was admitted to the hospital with stomachache, dizziness, vomiting, and fever, she had a severe infection and virtually no white blood cells. She died the next day.

• **Number two: Creating obstacles to reporting symptoms.** Patients frequently fail to report drug-induced side effects to their doctors.[13] That may be in large part because they don't even realize that their symptoms could be caused by a medication. If no one provides clear information about what to look for, potentially serious or even life-threatening side effects may be ignored until it is too late. Many health care providers don't encourage patients to report side effects or provide them an easy way to do so. These days, obstacles to clear communication, such as phone trees or overprotective receptionists, make it hard for patients to tell the doctor about drug-related side effects.

Why Patients May Not Report Side Effects

"Patients may not understand the significance of medication-related symptoms. They may be unsure if use of the medication in fact caused the symptom and may not want to seem like a hypochondriac. Patients may not want to bother the physician or communicate disappointing news about their failure to tolerate the therapy.... Patients may encounter obstacles to communication, such as delays on the telephone, difficulty in transmitting messages, or problems in scheduling timely office visits."[14]

From Weingart, S. "Patient-Reported Medication Symptoms in Primary Care," published in the *Archives of Internal Medicine*, 2005

• **Number three: Ignoring drug-induced symptoms.** Even when a patient suspects that a medication is causing serious problems and goes to an emergency department for medical attention, there is a strong probability that the doctors will fail to link drug-induced symptoms to medications 40 to 50 percent of the time.[15-16] Patients are frequently sent on their way without realizing that their medicine was responsible for their symptoms.

When a patient complains of dry mouth, dizziness, cough, memory problems, or muscle pain, it is easy to understand why the prescriber might be tempted to deny that the drug was at fault. Guilt is a powerful emotion, and no physician wants to believe she has harmed a patient. The inability or unwillingness to connect the dots to drugs demonstrates a fundamental weakness in medicine today.

• **Number four: Overriding medication alerts.** Patient safety experts all seem to agree on one thing: prescribing errors are common and frequently avoidable. Food and Drug Administration commissioner Margaret Hamburg, MD, stated in 2009, "I was stunned at the scope of the problem."[17]

So what does this mean for the average patient? One small study puts the problem of preventable adverse drug events into sharp focus. Researchers recruited 24 primary care physicians from the Boston area. Over the seven months of the study, these doctors wrote 2,134 prescriptions for the 661 patients who had agreed to participate. The results are truly amazing: "Of the 24 M.D. participants, 22 made at least one prescribing error over the seven-month period (92 percent) that led to a preventable or ameliorable ADE. The ADEs identified ranged in their degree of seriousness from minor events such as sleep disturbances to serious events such as gastro-intestinal bleeding."[18] It would not be unreasonable to conclude from these results that despite their good intentions, doctors often slip up and write a prescription that results in harm to the patient.

With so many errors linked to their prescribing patterns, you would think that most physicians would embrace technological tools like electronic prescribing that might reduce such mistakes. When a doctor prescribes a drug using her computer, smart phone, or PDA (personal digital assistant), there is often an electronic alert that warns about drug allergies, contraindications, or drug interactions for that specific patient. Think of it a little like the "idiot light" on the dashboard of your car. If there is a sudden drop in oil pressure or loss of coolant from your radiator, a red light comes on warning you about potential danger to your engine. It would be reckless to ignore such alerts.

So how do prescribers respond to the alerts they receive on their computers or handheld devices? In a word, abysmally. One study of 2,872 clinicians in three states examined more than 3 million electronic prescriptions. The investigators found that these health professionals ignored three-quarters of the drug allergy warnings. Perhaps even more disquieting, the prescribers dismissed 90 percent of the serious drug interaction warnings. The authors of the study concluded that "clinicians override most medication alerts, suggesting that current medication safety alerts may be inadequate to protect patient safety."[19] No one knows when a physician decides to overlook an electronic prescription warning, and there are no consequences unless the patient dies. Even then the cause of the problem may not be recognized.

There is no simple solution. J. Lyle Bootman, PhD, ScD, is Dean of the College of Pharmacy at the University of Arizona. He co-chaired the Institute of Medicine's investigation into medication errors. He advises consumers "to be aggressive in questioning doctors, nurses and pharmacists about their medications, whether they're watching over a hospitalized loved one or figuring out their own pills at home."[20]

Those least able to protect themselves are the most vulnerable to adverse drug events. Over half a million children experience drug complications each year.[21] Many occur in children under five years of age. Senior citizens are equally at risk. At least 16 percent are prescribed inappropriate medications that land them in the hospital.[22] Finally, cancer patients are extremely vulnerable to medication errors involving chemotherapy. Because these medications are so toxic, extra care is required. Sadly, there are way too many complications caused by the wrong dose, the wrong drug, or the wrong combination of medications. Researchers have concluded that "the oncology community needs to develop safer practices for ordering, dispensing, administering, and monitoring these medications."[23]

To help you better protect those you love or yourself, we have created a list of questions to ask your doctor whenever a new medicine is started. We suggest making a copy and giving it to your prescriber and pharmacist every time you receive a prescription.

Drug Safety Questionnaire

To the Doctor or Pharmacist:

I can take my medicine more safely if I know the answers to these questions. Thank you for your assistance.

Purpose of medicine:

Lab tests needed:

_____

Date:

Result:

_____

Date:

Result:

Name of medicine:

Brand: _____

Generic: _____

....

Dose: _____

When to take: _____am _____pm

....

Take medicine:

_____with food   _____an hour before or two hours after meals

....

Foods to avoid, if any:

....

Special precautions, if any:

....

Contraindications or situations when this drug might be inappropriate, if any:

....

Interacting medicines to avoid, if any:

....

Common side effects:

....

Serious symptoms:
(I should notify my doctor immediately at phone # _____)

....

Date to discontinue, if ever: _____

(Photocopy this page and take it to your health care provider)

• **Number five: Being oblivious to drug prices.** A wise consumer trying to determine which car to buy may turn to *Consumer Reports* to assess things like reliability, safety, fuel economy, performance, comfort and convenience, owner satisfaction, and price. Contrast that with pharmaceuticals. Most physicians don't really know how much the medicine they prescribe will cost their patients. This is not our opinion, but rather the conclusion of researchers who combed the medical literature to determine doctors' knowledge about medication costs.[24] These investigators analyzed 24 articles from the world's medical literature. They concluded that physicians are ignorant of costs and tend to underestimate the price of expensive medicines and overestimate the price of inexpensive ones.[25] The problem is that doctors prescribe and patients pay the bills. We can't think of another situation where someone else decides what you need without knowing how much it will cost and how well it works but expects you to pick up the tab without complaining. Can you imagine going to a restaurant and having the maître d' "prescribe" your dinner without consulting you on your preferences or the price of the meal? Not hardly.

Even people with insurance may have to shell out substantial co-pays for pills. Brand-name drug costs have skyrocketed. Medicare Part D (drug coverage for senior citizens) covers 75 percent of the first couple of thousand dollars in drug costs, but then there is the dreaded "donut hole." When someone enters this zone, he has to pay 100 percent of prescription drug costs out of pocket until total expenditures exceed $5,100. This requirement is in flux thanks to health care reform (seniors will get a discount once they enter the donut hole), but it still represents substantial payments from patients. If the doctor doesn't know how much you will have to spend on your medicine, you could both be in for a rude surprise.

• **Number six: Not knowing actual drug effectiveness.** If you are like most people, you have no idea how effective your medication actually is. What's scarier, neither does your doctor. Busy physicians rarely have time to scour the literature to find all the relevant articles about the medicines they prescribe. Instead they rely on the FDA's seal of approval to guarantee effectiveness. On the surface, this might seem reasonable. After all, the law states unequivocally that all medicines must be proved "safe and effective" before they can be sold on drugstore shelves. The trouble is that no one at the FDA has bothered to define the terms *safe* and *effective.*

If you buy a new car, you expect it to start every time you turn the key. If the vehicle breaks down on the way to the grocery store, you will have it towed back to the dealer and demand that it be repaired under warranty. Drugs, on the other hand, do not come with warranties, and they frequently fail.

Allen Roses, MD, spilled the beans in 2003. At the time he was an executive at GSK (GlaxoSmithKline), one of the world's largest drug companies. Dr. Roses was a leading proponent of genetically targeted drug therapy and was making his case at a scientific meeting. In doing so, however, he revealed that "the vast majority of drugs—more than 90 percent—only work in 30 or 50 percent of the people."[26]

To appreciate Dr. Roses's candor, one need look no further than antidepressant medications. Over 100 million prescriptions are written each year for drugs like citalopram (Celexa), escitalopram (Lexapro), fluoxetine (Prozac), paroxetine (Paxil), and sertraline (Zoloft). A 2010 review of multiple studies concluded that such drugs were helpful for severe depression, but when it comes to mild to moderate depression, the benefit of antidepressant medications "may be minimal or nonexistent."[27] In fact, they were no better than sugar pills for relieving the symptoms of the mild to moderate depression for which they are frequently prescribed.

This wasn't the first time researchers reached such a conclusion. An "analysis of 96 antidepressant trials between 1979 and 1996 showed that in 52 percent of them, the effect of the antidepressant could not be distinguished from that of placebo."[28] In 2008, Irving Kirsch, MD, and his colleagues reported that "the overall effect of new-generation antidepressant medications is below recommended criteria for clinical significance."[29] In other words, the majority of drug studies couldn't demonstrate that an antidepressant was better than a placebo.

The final disappointment came from a $35 million project funded by the National Institute of Mental Health. This STAR*D (Sequenced Treatment Alternatives to Relieve Depression) study revealed that only one in four patients actually recovered from depression after taking an antidepressant,[30] and that was with optimal clinical support. Had these patients received more typical treatment without psychosocial support, the investigators speculated that actual remission rates might have been in single digits. The bottom line is that antidepressant drugs are woefully inadequate, they frequently cause side effects, and yet millions of people are prescribed such medications every year.

A dedicated doctor who wades through the official FDA prescribing information to try to learn about the effectiveness of antidepressants like citalopram (Celexa), fluoxetine (Prozac) or sertraline (Zoloft) will discover phrases like "superior to placebo" for easing major depression. There is little information on mild to moderate depression, since the evidence is lacking that such drugs will be helpful. And when it comes to comparing an antidepressant like citalopram (Celexa) to venlafaxine (Effexor) or desvenlafaxine (Pristiq) to escitaloprom (Lexapro), forget it; no such information is available.

It's not just antidepressant medications that provide questionable benefits. The FDA-sanctioned prescribing information for drugs used to treat Alzheimer's disease, like donepezil (Aricept), suggests that there is some "improvement in cognitive performance" compared with a placebo. But a study published in the journal *Lancet* found that "no significant benefits were seen with donepezil (Aricept) compared with placebo in institutionalisation (42 percent vs 44 percent at 3 years) or progression of disability (58 percent vs 59 percent at 3 years). . . . Interpretation: Donepezil is not cost effective, with benefits below minimally relevant thresholds."[31]

Whether it's something relatively minor, like a fungus infection of toenails, or something far more serious, such as schizophrenia or cancer, the pharmaceuticals we have available leave a lot to be desired. Trying to determine the effectiveness of medications to treat dozens of conditions is incredibly difficult. Most health professionals have no good way to determine the actual benefits and risks of the drugs they prescribe or dispense.

• **Number seven: Relying on surrogate markers.** Doctors have been sold on "surrogate endpoints"—easily measured effects of a medication that seem to be related to the primary goal, even though the connection may be indirect. For example, lower cholesterol (a surrogate endpoint) is believed to mean a lower likelihood of a heart attack (the primary goal of the medication). It is a lot cheaper and easier for a drug company to demonstrate that a medication can move a number on a gauge or a lab test rather than show that it can actually save lives. We're talking about the big three: blood pressure, cholesterol, and blood sugar. Doctors have assumed that lowering your numbers will be good for your health. But, dear reader, the real point of lowering your numbers is not to improve a score but to actually reduce the risk of getting a heart attack or a stroke or of dying prematurely.

So here's another secret your doctor may not share: many of the drugs prescribed so enthusiastically for conditions such as hypertension, diabetes, and high cholesterol may not make a real difference in outcomes that matter, such as heart attacks, strokes, or death.

Here's a case in point—the beta blocker atenolol (Tenormin), which is used to treat hypertension: Beta blockers have been prescribed for over thirty years. This class of medication has an important role to play in treating chest pain (angina), heart failure, and certain irregular heart rhythms. If someone experiences a heart attack, beta blockers can reduce the likelihood of another one. There is, however, rising concern that beta blockers should not be first-line treatments for high blood pressure.[32-35]

Atenolol is one of the most popular beta blockers in the United States. Almost 40 million prescriptions were dispensed last year, mostly for hypertension. It does lower blood pressure. But a review of the most significant studies involving atenolol for controlling hypertension concluded that this drug was no better than a placebo in reducing the risk of heart attacks or death.[36] Some research even suggests that atenolol might *increase* the risk of strokes and death. One cardiologist stated unequivocally, "Atenolol should not be used in the treatment of hypertension."[37] We caution, though, that beta blockers should not be stopped abruptly.

Cholesterol is another example of a surrogate endpoint. Doctors and patients alike assume that lowering cholesterol will automatically lower the risk of heart attacks, strokes, and death. At last count, roughly 20 million people take cholesterol-lowering statin drugs like atorvastatin (Lipitor), lovastatin (Mevacor), pravastatin (Pravachol), rosuvastatin (Crestor), and simvastatin (Zocor). For people with existing heart disease, there seems to be a consensus that statins save lives. But three-quarters of the prescriptions written for statins in the United States are for people with elevated cholesterol but without clear evidence of heart disease.[38] Their doctors prescribe statins in an attempt to prevent problems down the road.

The wisdom of this approach has now been called into question. A meta-analysis of eleven clinical trials involving more than 65,000 people without heart disease produced no evidence that statins saved lives.[39] These people had elevated cholesterol levels and other risk factors for heart disease but were otherwise healthy. Statins lowered their bad LDL (low-density lipoprotein) cholesterol on average from 138 to 98. But, and it's a very big but, lowering this surrogate marker did not produce a measurable benefit by improving longevity.

Finally, we come to the third leg of the three-legged stool: blood sugar and diabetes. People with elevated blood glucose levels are more susceptible to cardiovascular problems. Two of the most serious complications of this disease are heart attacks and strokes. That's why doctors try hard to help patients with diabetes control their blood glucose levels with medicine.

When the diabetes drug Avandia (rosiglitazone) was first introduced in the United States in 1999, there was a lot of enthusiasm about this new medication. Within a short amount of time Avandia became one of the top-selling diabetes drugs in the country, bringing in billions annually to the manufacturer, GlaxoSmithKline. Doctors embraced Avandia because it was quite effective at lowering blood sugar (a surrogate endpoint). Unfortunately, there was no evidence that the drug would actually reduce the cardiovascular complications of diabetes. Most clinicians overlooked the fact that it raised bad LDL cholesterol.

The bubble burst on June 14, 2007, when an article appeared in the *New England Journal of Medicine* analyzing forty-two trials of Avandia. The authors concluded that rather than preventing heart attacks, the drug actually *increased* the risk of such events by 43 percent.[40] A firestorm of controversy erupted after the publication of this analysis. Many physicians had a hard time believing that they had prescribed a drug that might have caused the very thing they were trying to prevent. Since this landmark study, however, there have been other reports suggesting that Avandia increases the risk for heart attacks as well as congestive heart failure, weight gain (bad for diabetics), and fractures in women. Even so, three years later, 1 million prescriptions were still being written each year for Avandia.[41]

In spring of 2010, David Graham, MD, and his FDA colleagues published a study of Medicare patients that showed Avandia increased the risk for strokes, heart failure, and death.[42] He estimated that 48,000 senior citizens may have experienced heart attacks, strokes, and other cardiovascular nastiness over a ten-year span because they took Avandia instead of a different diabetes drug.[43] Add in younger patients, and the number could approach 100,000 or more. These are the deadly consequences of focusing on a short-term surrogate marker instead of heart attacks and survival.

• **Number eight: Not checking for drug interactions.** Millions of people suffer adverse drug reactions each year, and many occur because of bad drug combinations. There are thousands of potentially hazardous drug interactions, and no human being can keep more than a fraction in his or her memory. Doctors should not even try.

Every time a doctor writes a new prescription, he must take the time to look up the new drug together with every other medicine (and supplement) the patient is taking. There are numerous resources available, from books to online references such as Epocrates.com or MediGuard.org. Many of the electronic prescribing programs that doctors can use these days offer alerts when there is a potential drug interaction. The problem, however, is that doctors are often in a hurry. They may not stop to check for interactions. When an alert pops up on the screen, they may see it as a nuisance. Doctors frequently override or ignore such alerts.[44] That may be okay some of the time, but it can put the patient in harm's way.

• **Number nine: Not staying up to date on new research.** It is extremely difficult for a busy clinician to spend hours perusing the medical literature. Failing to keep up with drug research, however, can cause tremendous trouble. Here is a case in point: too much potassium can kill suddenly if it makes the heart beat erratically. There are a number of medications that can increase the risk of potassium buildup in the body. They include ACEI (angiotensin-converting enzyme inhibitor) and ARB (angiotensin II receptor blocker) blood pressure drugs such as irbesartan (Avapro), benazepril (Lotensin), olmesartan (Benicar), losartan (Cozaar), valsartan (Diovan), enalapril (Vasotec), fosinopril (Monopril), lisinopril (Prinivil, Zestril), telmisartan (Micardis), quinapril (Accupril), ramipril (Altace), as well as a different type of drug, spironolactone (Aldactone). At the time of this writing, more than 150 million prescriptions were filled for these drugs annually. That's a lot of people.

Normally, such medications do not cause problems if a doctor is monitoring potassium levels. But if a patient taking one of these drugs develops a urinary tract infection, there is a good possibility that she will receive an antibiotic such as TMP/SMZ (trimethoprim plus sulfamethoxazole). This popular antibiotic was dispensed over 20 million times in 2009. In combination with one of the blood pressure medications listed above, TMP/SMZ can raise potassium so high so fast that patients land in the hospital.[45] For some, cardiac arrest could occur with no prior warning. The reasons behind this deadly arrhythmia might go undetected. With so many people taking blood pressure medications and antibiotics, this is a very real threat. Doctors have other choices for treating urinary tract infections, but if they don't stay on top of the research, they may not realize how dangerous this combination could be.

• **Number ten: Not reporting drug problems to the FDA.** The only way that the Food and Drug Administration can learn about unexpected drug side effects and warn the medical community is if doctors take the time to submit a report. It is only after dozens or even hundreds of such reports start to pile up that the agency begins to pay attention. It can take years before the FDA discovers unusual or life-threatening side effects through this voluntary drug reporting system. For example, it took decades for the FDA to realize that the decongestant phenylpropanolamine (PPA) increased the risk of strokes. Serious dangers associated with the stop-smoking drug Chantix (agitation, hostility, depressed mood, suicidal thoughts, severe skin reactions, and trouble driving) were discovered through reports to the FDA's MedWatch system.

Chantix Reaction

"I'm a fifty-five-year-old wife, mother and nana of six. I was a closet smoker, two or three per day. My pharmacist was singing the praises of Chantix, so I decided to see my doctor and get a script. I followed the program to a T and quit.

"I started dreaming about deceased friends and relatives. I assured them I would be with them soon. I wasn't mad or sad, just flat, and I hated my husband. Everything he did annoyed me. I wanted to put a pillow over his face for about five minutes and put him out of my misery!

"One day my daughter called me to say, on behalf of all my kids, that I'd changed and they were wondering what was wrong. I hung up, picked up my car keys, and bought three bottles of sleeping pills and a packet of razor blades. I drove to a rural area and wrote a note saying my work here is done.

"Six days later I woke up in an intensive care unit surrounded by family. Last rites had been given as my family watched a ventilator breathe for me. The emotional pain I suffered cannot be put into words. It was a total nightmare."

Terri, December 9, 2009

Physicians should play a crucial role in detecting serious "postmarketing" adverse drug effects. The trouble is that they rarely do so.[46] One analysis of 37 studies found that only 6 percent of "new, rare or serious" adverse drug reactions were reported spontaneously to regulatory authorities.[47] Many physicians may see such submissions as anecdotes and unscientific. But without this information, doctors will not realize that others have suffered the same problems their patients are experiencing. Patients should encourage their physicians to submit reports of serious or unexpected reactions to MedWatch. Often the physician will have the best knowledge of all the relevant details and reports from doctors will be taken more seriously by regulators.

Because prescription medications cause so much disability and death and because there are so many avoidable errors, patients must be assertive. We have already provided a Drug Safety Questionnaire (see page 85) that we encourage you to take along to your doctor and pharmacist. In addition, be sure to ask your doctor pertinent questions. There may not be enough time for her to respond to each one in detail, but this information is too important to ignore. The list is available in a convenient format in the appendix on page 258.

Top 10 Questions to Ask Your Doctor When You Get a Prescription

1. Is there another way to treat my condition besides this drug?
2. What is the evidence that this drug will produce a meaningful outcome, not just change numbers on a test?
3. How likely am I to get a benefit from this medication?
4. What are the most common side effects?
5. What are the most serious side effects?
6. What symptoms require me to contact you immediately?
7. How can I get through to you promptly?
8. How long do I need to take this medication?
9. How should I take this drug—with food or without, morning or evening?
10. Are there any special instructions for stopping this medicine?

CHAPTER 7

DRUG INTERACTIONS CAN BE DEADLY

Serotonin is a critically important neurochemical that helps control mood and also plays a key role in appetite, sexual behavior, pain, sleep, and learning. Millions take SSRI (selective serotonin reuptake inhibitor) antidepressant medications such as citalopram (Celexa), escitalopram (Lexapro), fluoxetine (Prozac), paroxetine (Paxil), or sertraline (Zoloft), which work by regulating serotonin levels in the brain. But too much of this chemical can lead to serotonin syndrome, a potentially life-threatening condition. Many physicians have never heard of it and don't think to diagnose it.

Jane was a healthy fifty-five-year-old woman with a history of migraine headaches. They occurred only about two or three times a year, but they were overwhelming. Jane was initially prescribed a migraine medicine called sumatriptan (Imitrex) and later was switched to rizatriptan (Maxalt). The idea was that she would take the medicine at the very first sign of a migraine to try to abort an attack before it could get a foothold. About 80 percent of the time, the medication worked to short-circuit the migraine. If it didn't, Jane would have a full-blown migraine that incapacitated her.

One morning in July 2004, Jane got up as usual and took her morning medications, including an SSRI-type antidepressant called sertraline (Zoloft), which had been prescribed to prevent migraine attacks. She sat down at the kitchen table and started to sense the dreaded aura of a migraine coming on. She popped the Maxalt to try to head off the attack. Within a few minutes, Jane complained of not feeling right, and her husband helped her back to bed. Over the next twenty minutes, her speech became scrambled, and she couldn't articulate a thought. Then she stopped talking completely. Her husband called 911, and by the time the ambulance arrived, Jane was semiconscious. Her blood pressure was sky high—216/160—and her arms were beginning to flap around involuntarily. Because of the uncontrollable arm movements, the emergency crew had a hard time getting an IV (intravenous) line into her vein. When Jane arrived at the hospital, her temperature was 104 degrees Fahrenheit, and her arms and legs were moving uncontrollably. She was unconscious and unresponsive.

The doctors assumed she was having a stroke and ordered a CT (computerized tomography) scan of her brain. Even though Jane was unconscious, she was so agitated that the doctors had to paralyze her so they could do the CT scan. Even though the test did not show signs of a stroke, the doctors were so convinced Jane was having a stroke that they ordered a lumbar puncture, looking for blood in her spinal column that would prove a stroke. Results: again negative. A neurologist proposed encephalitis as the next-best bet to explain Jane's dire situation. Spinal fluid was sent for both bacterial and viral cultures. A second CT scan was performed, just in case they had somehow missed a stroke the first time. All tests came back negative. Over the next several days, Jane remained heavily sedated, intubated, and on a ventilator. At one point, her distraught husband had to consider the possibility that she was brain dead and that he might be asked to pull the plug.

Finally, after five days, Jane opened her eyes and was able to speak a few words. Once she was off the ventilator, they ran an MRI (magnetic resonance imaging) scan, but again it was negative for everything. In her husband's words, all the sophisticated tests came up empty—"zero, zip, nada." Then he started searching the medical literature himself. He located the ten most important symptoms of serotonin syndrome: confusion, agitation, myoclonus (involuntary muscle twitches or contractions), hyperreflexia (overactive reflexes), diaphoresis (excessive sweating), shivering, tremor, diarrhea, poor coordination, and fever. Patients with three or more of these symptoms are considered positive for serotonin syndrome. Jane had eight out of ten. She also had a heart arrhythmia (ventricular tachycardia) that can occur with this condition. Eight days after taking sertraline and rizatriptan, Jane was finally home, neurologically intact and back to normal, with orders from the doctor to avoid taking Zoloft and Maxalt together. Interestingly, the hospitalist (a physician who specializes in hospital medicine) had never heard of serotonin syndrome, and nobody—not the emergency room doctors, the neurologist, or the cardiologist—had even considered serotonin syndrome in their differential diagnoses. The cardiologist who treated Joe's mother, Helen, was also unaware of serotonin syndrome, the condition that led to her death.

When Jane was hospitalized, there were no warnings in the official prescribing information about the dangers of combining an SSRI-type antidepressant such as sertraline with a triptan-type migraine medicine like rizatriptan. It's no wonder Jane's doctors didn't consider this possibility. Two years later, the Food and Drug Administration (FDA) issued a "Warning on Combining Triptans and SSRIs or SNRIs (serotonin-norepinephrine reuptake inhibitors). The FDA has alerted health care professionals about a possible life-threatening condition that can occur when triptans (e.g., Imitrex) are taken concomitantly with SSRIs (e.g., Paxil and Prozac) or SNRIs (e.g., Cymbalta)."[1-2]

Fluoxetine (Prozac) was the first SSRI-type antidepressant approved to treat depression, in December 1987. Five years later, sumatriptan (Imitrex), the first triptan, got the green light for migraine therapy. Millions of people take such drugs. For fourteen years, a patient who showed up at a pharmacy with prescriptions for both Prozac and Imitrex would not have triggered any alarms. And yet we now know that such a combination could be life threatening. Far too frequently, dangerous drug interactions are discovered purely by accident, years after medications have been approved for sale. It is only after a certain number of bodies have stacked up that the problem *may* get the attention of the FDA. We emphasize *may* because there are almost assuredly interactions that have never been discovered that could be killing people although no one has recognized the danger.

Drug interactions that make headlines usually involve celebrities. When Anna Nicole Smith died in 2007, it was ruled an accidental drug overdose. In reality, it was the combination of an old-fashioned sedative, chloral hydrate, plus four different antianxiety agents (clonazepam [Klonopin], diazepam [Valium], lorazepam [Ativan], meprobamate [Miltown]); an antiseizure medication (topiramate [Topamax]); a muscle relaxant (methocarbamol [Robaxin]); and a highly sedating antihistamine (diphenhydramine). In 2009, Michael Jackson also died largely because of drug interactions. His physician gave him similar sedatives (benzodiazepines) and then added the coup de grace, an anesthetic called propofol that was injected intravenously. Added to the other drugs he had been given, it is hardly any wonder that Michael stopped breathing.[3]

The tragic stories of pop idols make news. When an older person taking five or six medicines dies from a bleeding ulcer, a stroke, or a fall, barely anyone notices, and health care providers are not surprised. They assume death was the result of old age or an underlying health problem such as diabetes or heart disease. How many of these deaths are attributable to bad drug combinations is anyone's guess, but research shows that many trips to emergency rooms are clearly caused by incompatible mixtures of medicines.[4-6] If physicians, pharmacists, and nurses were more vigilant, many medication misadventures could be prevented.

There is no organized system for detecting drug-drug, drug-food, or drug-herb interactions. As a result, much of what shows up in the medical literature or in the official prescribing information comes from case reports, the least scientific method for detecting problems. If a patient reports a problem while taking two or three medicines simultaneously, the physician may or may not take it seriously. If the doctor is motivated, she might submit the story as a case report to a medical journal or the FDA. Unless someone else decides to pursue the report, though, there is no good way to tell whether the interaction is mild, severe, or just a coincidence. Doubtless there are hundreds or even thousands of insignificant interactions listed in computer databases because of this haphazard system and countless more serious ones that have gone unrecognized.

Doctors' Knowledge of Drug Interactions

Doctors, like the rest of us, frequently don't know what they don't know. Even when a dangerous drug-drug interaction is well established, there is no guarantee that a physician will recognize it. This complex problem gets relatively little time and attention in medical school, and consequently many doctors don't make it a priority. Because of this lack of attention, we consider drug interactions one of the scariest and most common screwups in medicine today. We constantly receive letters and e-mail messages from people concerned about the long laundry list of medications an older relative is taking. Frequently, we discover a number of incompatible medications that work at cross-purposes or cause serious symptoms.

Too Many Meds!

Q. My mother is eighty-five and under the care of an internist, a cardiologist, and a neurologist. She has almost no energy and is quite depressed. She takes Aldactone, atenolol, Crestor, Diovan, hydrochlorothiazide, Lexapro, Miacalcin, Neurontin, Nexium, Nitro-Dur, Norvasc, Plavix, Rhinocort, Synthroid, and tramadol. In addition, she takes Aleve for arthritis pain and aspirin twice a day as needed. She is also on a nitro patch for her heart. Are there any conflicts with her medications?

Kathy, October 20, 2008

A. If we count over-the-counter pain relievers, your mother is taking seventeen different drugs. Some combinations could be life threatening. Taking aspirin, Aleve, and Plavix together could increase the risk of hemorrhage, including bleeding ulcers. Perhaps that is why the internist prescribed the acid-suppressing drug Nexium. The trouble is, Nexium and similar medicines may undo the anticlotting benefits of Plavix.

Taking tramadol, Lexapro, and Aleve together with Neurontin could lead to excessive drowsiness, so it is hardly any wonder your mom has no energy.

We're amazed she is moving at all. Lexapro and tramadol could increase the risk for serotonin syndrome and seizures.

Aleve could reduce the effectiveness of atenolol to lower blood pressure. Aleve may also increase the risk for kidney problems in combination with Aldactone. There are many other potential interactions, but the point is that the three specialists each prescribed medicines that may not play well together.

When doctors are tested on their knowledge about serious drug interactions, they often come up surprisingly short. One such study was conducted by mailing a survey to 12,500 prescribers.[7] Physicians, nurse practitioners, and physician assistants were included. Sadly, only 950 (7.9 percent) were willing to take the test, which involved analyzing fourteen different drug pairs for compatibility. Four of the pairs were absolutely inappropriate. Two were potentially problematic but might be prescribed together if carefully monitored, and eight drug pairs posed no interaction problem. Doctors were asked to categorize the drug pairs as "contraindicated," "may be used together but with monitoring," "no interaction," or "not sure." The prescribers were asked to restrict their use of drug references when answering the questionnaire, though, since this was a take-home test and relied on the honor system, there was no way to know if they refrained from "cheating." Regardless, the results were abysmal.

The prescribers classified less than half of the fourteen drug pairs correctly.[8] Only about one in five prescribers knew that it was absolutely inappropriate to combine the antianxiety agent alprazolam (Xanax) with the antifungal drug itraconazole (Sporanox) or that prescribing cimetidine (Tagamet) with warfarin (Coumadin) was contraindicated. Less than one in four realized that taking a drug called methotrexate (used to treat rheumatoid arthritis, psoriasis, and cancer) together with an antibiotic called cotrimoxazole (Bactrim, Septra) was also inappropriate. By any standard grading system, these physicians scored an F.

Even when physicians were allowed to use drug references when answering interaction questions, they still flunked. Another study that allowed such support revealed that prescribers correctly categorized drug-drug interactions only 44 percent of the time.[9]

Such failing grades on take-home tests give us pause, but they are, after all, merely questionnaires. How do doctors fare in the real world? In a small study of patient admissions to a university hospital emergency department, the emergency physicians identified only one-quarter of the potential drug interactions.[10] Another study found that emergency physicians did equally poorly when it came to recognizing drug-related complications.[11] If a teenager missed three-quarters of the questions on a driver's test, he would not get a license.

A Canadian study tracked a dangerous drug interaction between the antibiotic cotrimoxazole (Bactrim, Septra), which is often prescribed for urinary tract infections, and certain blood pressure pills called ARBs (angiotensin II receptor blockers) and ACEIs (angiotensin-converting enzyme inhibitors). These are widely prescribed drugs such as irbesartan (Avapro), olmesartan (Benicar), valsartan (Diovan), and enalapril (Vasotec), lisinopril (Prinivil, Zestril), or ramipril (Altace). When this antibiotic is taken with one of these blood pressure medications, potassium levels can go so high that they could trigger life-threatening complications. The researchers tracked over 100,000 people who had received prescriptions for these antihypertensive medications. More than one in ten had indeed received the dangerous combo.[12] Those who did were almost seven times more likely to be hospitalized for problems due to high potassium than people taking different antibiotics.

Computers to the Rescue?

In all fairness to physicians, no human could ever master even a tiny fraction of the more than 100,000 potential drug-drug interactions that have been identified.[13] That's why there are computers, handheld personal digital assistants (PDAs), and smart phones that have access to databases with drug interaction information. Unfortunately, many busy physicians just don't take the time to look up all the medications a patient is taking to check for interactions. In one survey, only 38 percent of physicians "consulted electronic references when they needed to learn more about drug-drug interactions."[14]

There is an even more disturbing trend, however. Physicians who submit their prescriptions electronically via a computer or smart phone are often forced to utilize an automatic drug interaction surveillance system, known as CPOE (computerized physician order entry). It is supposed to send an electronic alert to the doctor in the event of a potential prescribing problem. Sounds like a great idea, but in practice, there are some major problems.

Computers are not perfect. The drug interaction software is only as accurate and up to date as the programmers who create the database. One study found significant omissions in the system physicians relied on to determine dangerous drug interactions.[15] Far more worrisome, however, are prescribers who override the warning alerts. One researcher noted that "available evidence strongly suggests that this technology improves patient safety.[16-17] However, providers often override warnings, even those involving potentially life-threatening situations."[18-19]

Why in the world would a physician ignore or override an alert about a drug interaction? After all, an estimated 20 to 30 percent of the millions of adverse drug events that happen each year are caused by drug interactions.[20-21] Can you imagine a pilot ignoring a warning light about the landing gear or navigation system? We have sat on airplanes for long periods of time while maintenance workers fixed something mundane like a light in the bathroom. Even when it is a false alarm, pilots make sure the warning is fully checked, and they apologize for the delay. The passengers are usually grateful that everything is double-checked. Shouldn't a doctor be equally careful?

Physicians explain why they ignore alerts and override drug-drug interaction warnings this way: "alert fatigue." Many of the warnings that come up on the computer seem to have ambiguous clinical significance. In other words, doctors perceive many, if not most, of the alerts as insignificant or false alarms. Do you remember the story of the boy who cried wolf too many times? When the wolf really did show up, no one paid the boy any attention. Many doctors may also miss dangerous, or even deadly, drug-drug interactions because they get in the habit of overriding most computerized warnings. It's as if they run a red light and get away with it. So they do it again. After a while, running red lights becomes routine, unless there's an accident. Unfortunately, doctors may not learn about the consequences of ignoring warnings as many of the drug "accidents" go unrecognized and unreported.[22]

A study carried out at six Veterans Affairs (VA) medical centers reveals the scope of the problem. Data were collected on prescriber overrides of drug interaction alerts between July 1, 2003, and June 30, 2004. Over that year, there was a total of 291,880 drug-drug interaction overrides.[23] Shockingly, 72 percent of the overrides were for alerts considered "critical drug-drug interactions" by the VA experts who set up the system. Theoretically, the prescribers are supposed to document their reasons for ignoring the warning so a pharmacist can review it and approve moving forward with the prescription. More than half the time, however, there was "no reason provided" by the prescriber to justify ignoring a critical drug interaction alert.

If you think that's bad, consider that the VA has one of the most comprehensive safety systems in medicine. Most hospitals do not approach the VA's commitment to patient safety. You can bet that there is even less oversight in nursing homes,[24] outpatient clinics, and doctors' offices. If the VA has such a strikingly poor track record when it comes to protecting patients from critical drug-drug interactions, we shudder to imagine what the situation is like elsewhere.

The Pharmacy Safety Net?

In baseball, if a pitcher throws a wild pitch and it gets past the catcher, there is always the backstop to make sure the ball doesn't go too far astray. The same thing is supposed to be true when it comes to prescribing. If a physician exercises bad judgment and prescribes an inappropriate medication, then overrides the computerized warning system,

Interaction Prevention

Q. I was hospitalized recently for eighteen days and was afraid I might never get out alive because of carelessness.

I learned years ago always to make sure the provider of any prescriptions is aware I take Parnate, an MAO [monoamine oxidase] inhibitor. I always write it down on medical information sheets. When the admitting nurse came to my room, I gave her the information, too. She asked if I could take Demerol, and I told her no.

Two days later, I found out I had been receiving double doses of Demerol as an injection. I immediately asked my nurse to contact the doctor about this, since I knew they could interact. He didn't want to look up the information himself, so I suggested he contact the doctor who prescribed Parnate. When he refused to do so, I quickly dismissed him.

After being released, I wrote to the top hospital administrator. He checked around and sent me a letter saying we would not be billed. I'm grateful for that, but I wonder what would have happened if I hadn't raised a fuss.

A. The consequences of mixing Parnate (tranylcypromine) with Demerol (meperidine) may include agitation, seizures, fever, coma, or death. Doctors are advised to avoid this drug combination, but, as our reader discovered, they don't always double-check.

there should be a safety net at the pharmacy. Although it is true that pharmacists are very well trained and often catch mistakes, the system is not foolproof. Pharmacists, like physicians, rely on their computers to catch drug interaction problems. But, as we have already noted, not all computerized databases are complete and up to date. In addition, pharmacists and pharmacy techs also override drug interaction alerts for much the same reason that doctors do: they perceive many warnings as either a nuisance, clinically insignificant, or a false alarm.

Frustrated Clinical Pharmacist

"A patient presented to our pharmacy with four prescriptions from an urgent care center. The prescriptions were written for citalopram, tramadol, prednisone, and clonazepam. As there is a drug-to-drug interaction with citalopram and tramadol I faxed the prescriber the following note: 'drug-to-drug interaction citalopram + tramadol per official compendia checked' (I named the references). 'Increased risk of serotonin syndrome, increased seizure risk. Please advise and thanks.'

"The prescriber faxed back the same four prescriptions on the same prescription blank with citalopram crossed out and fluoxetine prescribed instead. I was flabbergasted. Did he really not know that citalopram and fluoxetine are in the same class of drugs, SSRIs? At this point, I had to fax him back *again* to inform him that 'all SSRIs interact with tramadol, and what needs to be changed is the pain medication.'

"The prescriber never got back to us, so the tramadol still sat in our 'problem' area. It could not be filled because of the drug interaction.

"Fast-forward to the following day. The patient showed up to pick up his prescriptions, but the pain medication issue was still not resolved. I discussed the problem with the patient. I asked him why the drugs were prescribed, and he said he was being treated for a back problem. He indicated that the prescriber was considering propoxyphene for pain instead of tramadol. I explained that propoxyphene has the same potential for interacting with his antidepressant, citalopram.

"It took many phone calls that were handled by the receptionist for this patient to get the medicine he needed for safe control of his back pain. We spent a lot of time getting this right. We do not have time for prescribers who are not knowledgeable about medication therapy and who do not think enough of either their patients or other health care professionals to actually speak to us themselves. The ridiculous game of 'medicine by receptionist' should be discontinued. But pharmacists have no choice. We are the last professional patients see before they put the medication in their body, and it is imperative that it be correct."

Even when the pharmacist catches a critical drug-drug interaction and calls the doctor's office, the physician may not return the call. At other times, a receptionist or nurse in the doctor's office might approve the prescription without checking to make sure it is really safe. Pharmacists have also shared stories about doctors who became angry when a pharmacist called with a concern about a potential drug interaction.

Overlooking Interactions

"My wife has been treated for multiple sclerosis for more than three years. She had all sorts of tests. Despite treatment, my wife had serious problems—falling and even passing out.

"All doctors she saw (at least seven of them, including specialists at a teaching hospital) looked at the list of medications she was taking and said nothing about any incompatibilities. After all of this time, we visited another doctor who looked at the medication list and was alarmed about Pamelor, a drug that my wife had taken for about four years. A blood test showed the blood level of this drug was in the toxic range. She stopped it immediately, and all the problems we had agonized over for so long were gone.

"We get all of our medications from the same pharmacy, and they *did* question this medication as interacting with another she was taking. The pharmacist called the doctor and he said it was okay. Now we know that the pharmacist was right to question this combination. I just can't believe that we saw so many different doctors during this period, all had the same list of medications, and none of them spotted the problem."

You cannot assume your prescriber has taken the time to check for incompatible combinations. There is a distinct possibility that your physician might ignore or override warnings about interactions. Even if your pharmacist catches a mistake, your doctor may choose to ignore it. That means that you and your family are going to have to take a very active role in managing the medications you take.

Top 11 Tips for Preventing Dangerous Drug Interactions

1. **Take a list of all your medicines to your appointment.** If this is too complicated, put all your bottles into a brown bag and take them along. Make sure to include vitamins, dietary supplements, herbs, and over-the-counter medications. Make sure the entire list is entered into your electronic medical record and reviewed again before any prescription is written.

2. **Find out how to take your medicine!** Always ask your prescriber how to swallow your pills—what time of day, on an empty stomach, or with meals. Write this information down and then double-check with the pharmacist without revealing what the doctor told you. This will give you independent verification about how to take your medicine.

3. **Check about whether any foods or beverages should be avoided.** A surprising number of drugs can interact with grapefruit juice, for example. Several important medicines won't work as expected if taken with calcium-fortified orange juice. Even apple juice can alter how some drugs are absorbed and metabolized.

4. **Ask your doctor to check for interactions.** Before you leave the office, verify that your physician has reviewed your entire list of drugs and dietary supplements to make sure there are no incompatible combinations. If your doctor is using a computer or handheld device to submit your prescription electronically, ask if there are any drug interaction alerts that you should know about.

5. **Ask your pharmacist to check for interactions.** Do not grab and go when you pick up your prescription. Instead, ask to speak with a pharmacist. Inquire whether there were any interaction alerts that came up on your record. If so, find out what they were. Even if the pharmacist says they were not important, you need to have a written

record of potential problems. While you are at it, ask about food-drug interactions as well. See if the information you get from the pharmacy agrees with what the doctor told you.

6. **Inquire about over-the-counter drugs.** Your pharmacist is more likely to know about potential drug interactions between your prescription and over-the-counter pills than the prescriber. Even heartburn medicine like cimetidine (Tagamet) or omeprazole (Prilosec), as well as pain relievers such as aspirin, ibuprofen, or naproxen, may sometimes interact dangerously with prescription medications.

7. **Go to the Web to check on interactions yourself.** The best resource we know of is MediGuard.org (www.Mediguard.org). This website allows you to enter all your medicines, including supplements, as well as your conditions. It will give you a detailed report on potential interactions. This free service is well worth the time and is likely to be more up to date than other databases.

8. **Don't take herbs or dietary supplements without checking for interactions.** Many people assume that natural products are completely safe. They also fear that their provider will look askance if they admit to taking unconventional products. This is risky business. Many herbs can interact with prescription medications. St. John's wort is a classic example. Even the spice turmeric (curcumin), used to treat arthritis and psoriasis, may interact dangerously with several prescription drugs. You may find some information about herb-drug interactions at MediGuard.org, or you might ask your pharmacist to refer you to someone who is knowledgeable.

9. **Beware drug-alcohol interactions.** Many prescribers fail to mention that alcohol may interact with a prescription drug. Some drugs can actually increase blood levels of alcohol. Even modest alcohol consumption could result in intoxication. Alcohol can also affect how your body handles a medication.

10. **Inquire about drug-disease interactions.** Some medications can make certain conditions worse. For example, beta blockers used to treat high blood pressure or heart problems can aggravate asthma. Cholesterol-lowering statins can occasionally raise blood sugar levels, making diabetes control more complicated.

11. **Check for prescription drug effects on laboratory test results.** Some medications alter test results and give false positives or false negatives. For example, women who take birth control pills or hormone replacement therapy may not get an accurate reading on their total T_4 test, which may be falsely elevated. This measure of thyroid function might mislead the prescriber if drug-lab interactions are not considered.

CHAPTER 8

TOP 10 SCREWUPS PHARMACISTS MAKE

1. Not counseling patients
2. Dispensing the wrong drug
3. Dispensing the wrong dose
4. Ignoring interactions
5. Not standing up to doctors
6. Trusting all generic drugs
7. Relying on inadequate labels and leaflets
8. Not reporting errors
9. Switching drugs without patient approval
10. Not supervising techs carefully

Drugstore Disasters

Most pharmacists are incredibly well trained. They graduate with a Doctor of Pharmacy (PharmD) degree. That means they spend two to four years in an undergraduate college program plus an additional four years in a pharmacy school. There are a licensure exam and continuing education requirements. The training is rigorous and expensive, but it pays off. A comprehensive survey shows that the average pharmacist receives $115,455 a year (roughly $55 per hour), not including the bonus, which averages over $5,000.[1]

Contrast that with pharmacy technicians. There are "no standard training requirements," and, in many states, not even a high school diploma is necessary.[2] Some do get training at a community or technical college, but many get in-house or on-the-job training from their employer. It comes as a shock to most people to learn that pharmacy technicians are not uniformly trained and certified. They generally make anywhere from about $10 to $16 an hour.[3]

Many customers don't even realize that the person who hands them their prescription usually knows virtually nothing about the medicine. Because techs and pharmacists both wear white coats, it can be difficult to determine at a glance who's the professional and who's the low-paid assistant. But asking a pharmacy tech a question about your medicine could be a bit like asking a baggage handler to fly an airplane.

Nonetheless, in many busy pharmacies, the techs actually prepare many of the prescriptions. Pharmacists are supposed to check them carefully, but a tragic mistake made by a tech led to the death of a toddler named Emily Jerry. She was given an injection for cancer treatment that contained so much sodium that it killed her. The supervising pharmacist was too busy to catch the error. This incident inspired legislation introduced in Congress in 2008 ("Emily's Act"). The bill noted that in 2006, the Joint Commission that accredits hospitals found that hospital pharmacists caught about 80 percent of the mistakes their technicians made.[4] That means one out of five mistakes could have slipped through the cracks, and almost a quarter of them could have caused serious harm. There is a good chance that community pharmacists catch even fewer errors.

The typical busy chain pharmacy is a pressure cooker, filling more than 250 prescriptions each day, and some dispense considerably more. One insider likened the process to a fast-food restaurant where the emphasis is on serving up as many burgers as possible in the shortest amount of time. They are filling scripts as fast as they can while being distracted by phone calls from doctors' offices, patients, and insurance companies. They also have to deal with drive-through windows, just as at a fast-food restaurant. We frequently hear from pharmacists that they don't have time to eat lunch or take a bathroom break.

This kind of work environment is a breeding ground for errors. According to a 2003 study, the average pharmacy fills four prescriptions incorrectly each day. The researchers estimated that this would add up to 51.5 million errors annually.[5] Most of the mistakes were relatively minor, but many could affect patients' health.

A more recent study (2009) carried out with trained secret shoppers uncovered an even higher rate of mistakes. One out of five prescriptions dispensed deviated from the physicians' written orders.[6] If you extrapolate 20 percent of the approximately 4 billion prescriptions filled in the United States each year, you end up with as many as 800 million pharmacy mistakes annually.

Can you wrap your mind around that number? We can't. Even if the number were only one-tenth that size, it would still be *80 million* errors each year. No other industry would be allowed to make so many mistakes year in and year out. (A similar dispensing error rate was revealed fourteen years earlier.[7]) Of course, not all these errors are life threatening, but about 3 percent were considered "potentially harmful."[8] Extrapolating, that means 24 million prescription errors each year could represent a health problem for patients. Don't let someone you care about become a victim!

Top 10 Pharmacist Screwups

• **Number one: Not counseling patients.** The whole reason pharmacists spend so many years learning about drugs is to protect patients. They should not have to "count, pour, lick, and stick." That used to describe the dispensing duties of pharmacists as they moved pills from big bottles into little ones. Go back far enough, though, and you would find that pharmacists usually had time to talk to people, give advice, and help solve simple health problems. No wonder they were often called "doc."

These days, few patients speak directly to the pharmacist. The clerk or the pharmacy tech shoves a sheet of paper at the customer for her to sign, waiving the right to pharmacist counseling. According to one study, the rate of counseling has dropped nearly by half, from 43 to 27 percent, over the past fourteen years.[9] The secret shopper study mentioned previously found that pharmacists offered counseling for new prescriptions only about one-quarter of the time.[10] Customers have a right to the valuable information pharmacists have to offer, so be sure to ask to speak with a pharmacist about how to take your medicines and what side effects to watch out for. Pharmacists should use the teach-back technique to make sure their clients understand the counseling they give.

• **Number two: Dispensing the wrong drug.** Drug names that look alike or sound alike—such as Lamictal and Lamisil or Zantac and Xanax—are easily confused. Whenever a medicine is called in or faxed from a doctor's office, the chances for mistakes are increased substantially.

Never assume that the pills in your bottle are the right ones. Just as you count the money that a bank teller or an ATM (automated teller machine) gives you, you should look at the label on the prescription and check to make sure the patient's name, the drug name, and the dose all correspond to the prescription the doctor wrote. For that reason, it is handy to keep a photocopy of the prescription before you give the original to the drugstore. If it is a refill, open the bottle, and make sure the pills look the same. If they don't, ask the pharmacist about it. A different generic formulation may well be a different size or color without posing a problem, but having the pharmacist look the prescription over one last time before you take it home is not such a bad idea.

Deadly Pharmacy Mistake

In 2002, a seventy-nine-year-old man named Leonard Kulisek was wrongly given glipizide, a diabetes medicine, instead of the drug his doctor had prescribed for gout. The glipizide caused kidney toxicity that ultimately led to his death.[11]

• **Number three: Dispensing the wrong dose.** Many medications come in a wide range of doses. Your doctor hopefully had a good reason to believe that the dose she prescribed would be the right one for you. Make sure it is the one you get. You would be amazed how many times dosing errors occur and lead to serious harm, if not death. This is even more important in the hospital. Check every single medication that is dispensed, and make sure the person who administers a drug verifies the dose of all oral and injectable medicines each time.

Deadly Dosing Error

Beth Hippely received a prescription for the blood thinner Coumadin (warfarin) that was ten times higher than she had been prescribed. As a result, she suffered a bleeding stroke that left her severely disabled.[12]

• **Number four: Ignoring interactions.** Pharmacists are supposed to catch doctors' mistakes when it comes to interactions. In fact, the pharmacist may be the only professional who can keep track of all the medications a patient has been prescribed. These days, it is not unusual for a person to see several specialists in addition to a primary care provider. These prescribers rarely communicate with one another, especially with regard to medications.

Today's modern pharmacy comes equipped with computers to help the pharmacist dispense and label drugs efficiently. They also flag potential drug interactions. And therein lies the dilemma. Warnings about routine interactions can be overridden by a pharmacy tech who knows virtually nothing about such incompatibilities. If warnings pop up too often, they lose their impact. When interactions are ignored, however, the patient may be put at risk.

Before dispensing a medication that could prove dangerous when combined with other medicine, the pharmacist must contact the prescriber. This is far easier said than done. Here's a deadly secret neither doctors nor pharmacists are likely to share: not all doctors return pharmacy calls promptly. It can take hours or days for a busy practitioner to call the pharmacy back. Some calls are never returned. If you are waiting to pick up your medicine, this can be maddening. Even worse, some physicians are offended when a pharmacist questions a prescription. It's little wonder that pharmacists may be tempted to dispense a drug without ruffling feathers, despite concerns about patient safety.

So how well do pharmacists protect patients from dangerous or deadly drug interactions? Not well enough. In one study, secret shoppers were sent to 245 pharmacies in seven cities around the country. They submitted two incompatible prescriptions at the drugstore counter, and at least one-third of the time they were given both drugs without a warning.[13]

In another study, secret shoppers submitted a prescription for the blood thinner warfarin (Coumadin). This drug should never be taken with aspirin unless the doctor is monitoring blood coagulation very carefully, and no pharmacy should ever sell aspirin with warfarin. In this investigation, however, more than two-thirds of the shoppers were able to buy over-the-counter aspirin at the same time they picked up their warfarin and got no warning at all.[14] Bottom line: do not assume your pharmacy will catch all the important drug interactions you should know about. Do your own homework. One place to check is www.MediGuard.org.

• **Number five: Not standing up to doctors.** Pharmacists are one of the most respected professionals, ranking above physicians in the minds of the American public. Sadly, though, many physicians don't see it that way. Sometimes doctors make it clear that they know best, even when they prescribe the wrong dose or the wrong combination of pills. Pharmacists who call a doctor to ask a question or politely point out an error are sometimes chastised. Just getting past the receptionist can be a challenge, if not impossible. That policy comes straight from the doctor, since most physicians don't delay in taking calls from their medical colleagues. The pharmacist is legally liable for dispensing a dangerous combination or dose. That's why it is essential for pharmacists to always be assertive in dealing with doctors if they suspect a safety problem for a patient.

• **Number six: Trusting all generic drugs.** We were big boosters of generic drugs for twenty-five years, starting even before most pharmacists got on board with the program. There is no question that they save money. Now everyone who pays for prescriptions loves generics, including insurance companies and the federal government. Pharmacies get a good deal on many generics and can sometimes enjoy a decent markup.

There is a fly in the ointment, however. Starting about ten years ago, we discovered that the approval process the Food and Drug Administration (FDA) has put in place for generic medications has flaws. Even worse, the FDA doesn't have the resources to monitor the manufacturing process adequately, especially in overseas plants. In recent years, we have seen problems with numerous generic drugs, and there have been an astonishing number of recalls. Pharmacists who insist that all generic drugs are identical have not been paying attention. When a patient finds that a particular generic does not work or is causing complications, the pharmacist ought to investigate with an open mind. Blindly accepting the FDA's assertion that all generic drugs are "identical" is not in the patient's best interests.

Generic Drug Equivalence Issues

"My wife had done well on the brand-name antidepressant Wellbutrin XL 300 and then the Watson generic bupropion for several years. She was abruptly switched to Teva Budeprion last spring. Gradually, her depression returned. It was as if she were taking a placebo. Within a month, she was on the brink of suicide.

"When I realized how severe her situation was, I ran out and purchased brand-name Wellbutrin. It took less than a week for her to return to her normal cheerful self."

G.I., February 2009

• **Number seven: Relying on inadequate labels and leaflets.** Pharmacists have very little room on a prescription bottle to provide instructions and warnings. You actually get a lot more information on over-the-counter medications than you do with your prescription.

Tiny labels with hard-to-read print may tell you to take your pills before meals or to avoid dairy products. But unless you have spoken with the pharmacist (see mistake number one), it's almost impossible to say whether "take before meals" means half an hour, a couple of minutes, or an hour. These seemingly subtle nuances can actually have a big impact on drug effectiveness.

You do get a bit more precision, seemingly, if you read the printed leaflet that often comes with your medicine. But you might be surprised to learn that the information in these handouts varies quite a bit from one drug chain to the next. They are not always kept up to date with the latest side effect or interaction facts. An evaluation of such leaflets found in 384 community pharmacies in forty-four states concluded that four-fifths did not have specific directions, and one-quarter had hard-to-read print. The authors concluded, "Fewer than 10 percent of all leaflets met quality criteria regarding contraindications, precautions, and how to avoid harm."[15]

• **Number eight: Not reporting errors.** Pilot error is scrutinized closely; when airplane pilots have a "near miss," they are expected to report it immediately. Even if there is no accident, federal regulators and fellow pilots want to know so that they can help prevent similar problems in the future.

Pharmacists, however, don't have to report near misses or even serious mistakes. Dispensing the wrong drug or the wrong dose of a drug to a patient triggers no report or action. There is no federal or state organization set up to even receive such a report. At the time of this writing, only the state of North Carolina consistently requires pharmacists to report errors that lead to deaths. Given the magnitude of the problem (an estimated 800 million mistakes annually), it is hardly any wonder that nothing is being done, since no one is keeping track. The only way to improve this dismal situation is to require that reports of mistakes be filed with a national organization that can ultimately make recommendations to stop this epidemic of errors.

• **Number nine: Switching drugs without patient approval.** You would think that if a physician determines the best medication for a patient, that's the drug the patient would receive. There would be no quibbling or switching. You would be wrong. Pharmacists frequently substitute a generic drug for a brand name without even a second thought. Unless the doctor specifically writes something like "dispense as written" or "do not substitute," you may get a generic even if your doctor has prescribed the brand-name version. During the switch, there is often room for a slipup.

Even more alarming, however, is the practice of "therapeutic substitution." In some states, pharmacists can switch a patient from one drug to another in the same category, especially if the insurance company requests it. For example, your doctor might prescribe Lipitor to lower your cholesterol. The pharmacist might fill that with simvastatin (also known as Zocor) instead. In most cases, that substitution won't cause problems. But substituting can sometimes lead to dreadful consequences. A postal carrier we know was doing well on brand-name Zantac for reflux back when it was a prescription drug. The pharmacist substituted generic cimetidine (the generic form of Tagamet) at the request of the insurance company. The result was a life-threatening skin reaction called Stevens-Johnson syndrome that landed him in the hospital for weeks. Do not accept a switch unless you and your doctor have approved it.

• **Number ten: Not supervising techs carefully.** As we explained earlier, there is a huge gap between the education required of pharmacists and that required for pharmacy technicians. The system is set up on the assumption that the pharmacist will be more or less looking over the tech's shoulder and checking his or her work at all times. That certainly happens in many pharmacies, but the level of supervision can be quite variable. We have personally witnessed technicians filling and dispensing prescriptions with minimal oversight. Imagine the outrage if dental hygienists started filling cavities or performing oral surgery.

Research shows that in a hospital setting, pharmacists fail to catch one out of five technician errors.[16] We suspect that pharmacists in large chain drugstores might be even less vigilant. Nursing homes that use technicians to give out medications also seem to have a high medication error rate.[17] What happens in huge, mail-order pharmacy operations, where everything is highly automated, is anyone's guess.

MD and Mail-Order Mess-Up!

In May 2010 we received the following question from a listener to our radio show:

"I receive my medication from a mail-order pharmacy service. I have been taking the medication gabapentin (600 mg four times a day). I just received a bottle of Neurontin (600 mg) with instructions to take two pills four times a day. Is this new dose correct?"

Of course there was no way for us to know the correct answer. Neurontin is the brand name, and gabapentin is the generic form of this epilepsy drug. Clearly, there was a slipup somewhere during the switch from generic to brand name. The normal dose of this medicine ranges from 900 mg to 1800 mg a day. The dose our listener was initially taking, 2400 mg, was at the high end of the acceptable range. The new dose (4800 mg) was substantially outside of the norm. We encouraged this person to contact both the mail-order pharmacy and the physician to find out what went wrong. Here is what she found out.

"It took quite a while on hold, but I talked to a pharmacist at the mail-order center. She said the dose was what was on the prescription, and she guessed that it was probably correct because that is not an uncommon dosage. After two days, I received a call back from the doctor's office. They admitted they had made a mistake and sent in the wrong dosage. If I had taken the double dose, I would still be sleeping."

We wanted to confirm that the doctor's office had incorrectly doubled the dose and that the mail-order pharmacy had missed the mistake. Symptoms of such a high dose would likely have been drowsiness, dizziness, unsteadiness, lethargy, nausea, and diarrhea. Our listener responded:

"Yes, the doctor's office admitted they had doubled the dose in error. The mail-order pharmacist not only did *not* catch the mistake but said that dose was fine and a common dosage. It just goes to show that we the people have to be responsible for educating ourselves about our health and well-being in all matters."

T. F., May 2010

CHAPTER 9

GENERIC DRUG SCREWUPS

Everyone loves a bargain. When we see 20 percent off on our favorite paper towels, we enthusiastically snap them up. If we find a big sale on chicken, we promptly add it to our cart. People travel long distances to outlet malls to save 30 to 50 percent on brand-name products. Seeking high quality for less money is as American as apple pie.

But all these efforts pale in comparison to the savings that can be achieved by buying generic drugs instead of brand names. That's because a basic law of economics has been suspended. We've all heard the expression "You get what you pay for." That's why some people are willing to pay extra for Dole pineapple or Godiva chocolate. We recognize that if someone tries to sell us a "Rolex" watch for $312 that normally costs $12,027, the chances are good it is either stolen, a "replica," or counterfeit. We should not expect a cheap knock-off watch to keep time or last like a Rolex that costs roughly forty times as much.

In the world of pharmaceuticals, however, we are told that, regardless of the price we pay, generic drugs are "identical" to their brand-name counterparts. For example, a three-months' supply of Mevacor, which lowers cholesterol, would normally cost over $250. The FDA assures us that the generic version lovastatin that we can buy at a big-box discount drugstore for $10 is absolutely the same. Ditto for a ninety-day supply of Prozac, which costs a little over $600. The same quantity of a generic form of fluoxetine is supposed to be the absolute equal of the brand-name Prozac. In other words, we can save $590 (98 percent) and have a duplicate drug.

Prozac Predicament

"I am a psychiatrist in private practice and have had three patients in the last few months have problems with generic Prozac (fluoxetine). The reports are consistent—lost efficacy and sedation where there had been none on the brand name. One patient experienced withdrawal symptoms after missing a dose, which should not happen with fluoxetine, given its long half-life.

"I went so far as to try both the generic and the Eli Lilly Prozac myself. I would agree, based on side effects, that they were not only different strengths but different drugs. The generic appears to be a short-acting, sedating weak-dose SSRI [selective/serotonin reuptake inhibitor] (perhaps paroxetine or fluvoxamine rather than fluoxetine).

"All three patients improved within two weeks on brand-name Prozac with resolution of all side effects."

October 15, 2007

Let's put this in another context. Say you decided to buy a new laptap computer from Dell. At the time of this writing, you could purchase a Dell Inspiron 15R for $599.99. If you were told you could purchase a brand-new identical computer that would perform precisely the same way the Dell Inspiron 15R does for $10, you would assume it was a scam.

How is it that we can pay so little for generic drugs and still get perfect quality? The answer, we are told, is that generic drug companies do not have to pay for research and development (R&D). Since a big part of the price of brand-name medicine comes from R&D, the generic manufacturers can presumably save us gobs of money without sacrificing quality. All they have to prove to the Food and Drug Administration (FDA) is that their medicine gets into the bloodstream in a manner similar to that of the brand name so it can be considered "bioequivalent."

What Are Generic Drugs?

In answering the question "What are generic drugs?" on its website, the Food and Drug Administration states unequivocally:

"A generic drug is identical—or bioequivalent—to a brand name drug in dosage form, safety, strength, route of administration, quality, performance characteristics and intended use."[1]

The FDA's definition of *identical* is quite different from normal folks. If you check the Oxford Dictionary, you will find this definition for the word *identical*:

adj. 1 agreeing in every detail. 2 one and the same.

The *Merriam-Webster Unabridged Collegiate Dictionary* defines *identical* as

1: being the same 2: having such close resemblance as to be essentially the same.

Given such definitions, it's only logical that patients, physicians, and pharmacists would assume that all generic drugs are exactly the same as their brand-name counterparts. The reality, however, is not so clear. The FDA does not require generic drugs to contain the same inactive ingredients as the brand-name product. Colors, binders, and fillers that often make up most of the content of the pills can be quite different. This could mean that someone is allergic to one formulation of a generic even though he tolerates the brand name or a different generic. As you will read shortly, the way pills are designed to release their active ingredients can also differ substantially from brand to generic drug. That is not our understanding of the word *identical*.

Promoting Generic Drugs

We believed the FDA's generic story for more than twenty-five years. In fact, when our first book, *The People's Pharmacy,* was published in

1976, we castigated physicians and pharmacists for not prescribing and dispensing more generic drugs.[2] In those days, generics were a relatively small percentage of the dispensed drugs in America, and most were made in the United States. The FDA actually tested batches of antibiotics from each manufacturer before the products could be released for market. Whenever questions about quality arose, we staunchly defended the FDA's system for approving and monitoring generic drugs.

Throughout the 1990s, we continued to promote generic drugs and to defend the FDA. We were, however, beginning to wonder whether our unquestioning enthusiasm was justified. In June 1998, a nurse with eighteen years' experience in a cardiologist's office maintained that she had seen several cases in which the generic anticoagulant warfarin was not equivalent to brand-name Coumadin. That same year, we heard from a patient with a sluggish thyroid gland: "I have been treated for hypothyroidism for over thirty years and have been on Synthroid 0.125 mg for the past ten. This year, my doctor wrote the prescription for a generic at the same dose. By the fourth day on the generic, I felt as though I was on the end of a tightly coiled spring. I couldn't sleep, I had a slight case of diarrhea, I was sweating more than usual, and my heart felt as though it would pound out of my chest. When I finally realized all this might be due to the change in medication, I had the pharmacist give me Synthroid instead. Almost immediately, I calmed down, my heart stopped pounding so hard, and I was back to my normal self. Why should this drug have affected me so?"

We had no good answer, but all the symptoms this person reported were suggestive of an excessively high dose of thyroid hormone. Our doubts were getting stronger because we were starting to receive more complaints from other patients. Still we refrained from questioning the FDA's oversight. This was at a time when most other health professionals—physicians, pharmacists, and nurses—were embracing generics with our old enthusiasm. Insurance companies, hoping to save money, were encouraging (or forcing) people to switch to generics whenever possible. Over two decades, generics had increased to almost 50 percent of all dispensed prescriptions; today, generic drugs have captured over 70 percent of the market. Something else was beginning to happen. Generic companies were outsourcing production to foreign countries.

Lasix vs. Generic Furosemide

The diuretic Lasix (furosemide) is a critically important drug for people suffering congestive heart failure. Inadequate dosing can have devastating consequences.

"My brother was taking Lasix and later was given furosemide. This almost killed him because he did not get rid of the water in his body as he had with Lasix. My mother-in-law suffered a very similar situation on furosemide. I also had the same reaction, as did my cousin. They tell the people the generic is the same, but I know for a fact that furosemide is not the same. This is dangerous to give to people who need Lasix!"

Anonymous, April 9, 2007

Investigating the FDA

By 2002, our concerns about generic drug quality had reached a tipping point because of ever-increasing consumer complaints. We started investigating the FDA's oversight of the generic marketplace, and what we discovered astonished us. For one thing, there was no centralized monitoring system. FDA's Office of Generic Drugs seemed to have one primary goal: approve generic drugs as quickly as possible. Once generics were on the market, there was virtually no further oversight from that group. At that time that fell to the Postmarket Surveillance Team in the Division of Prescription Drug Compliance at the Center for Drug Evaluation and Research for the FDA. We talked to the team leader, Jay Schmid.[3]

In 2002, we learned that the FDA tested about 50 or 60 different brand and generic drugs off pharmacy shelves each year. The agency actually analyzed about three hundred "finished dosage forms" of those fifty or sixty different drugs; that was out of roughly 3 billion prescriptions. In other words, the FDA actually checked on 0.00001 percent of the drugs dispensed from retail pharmacies, or 1 out of 10 million. And that didn't take into account all the drugs dispensed from hospitals, HMOs, the VA, or nursing homes.

It dawned on us that the FDA mostly relies on the honor system when it comes to monitoring both generic and brand-name drugs. Although inspectors are supposed to visit each drug manufacturing plant every two years, the agency doesn't have the manpower or resources to accomplish this task. Nicholas Buhay, then deputy director of the Division of Manufacturing and Product Quality at the FDA, admitted to us in 2002 that the fifty inspectors devoted to visiting generic drug plants can't visit all manufacturing facilities in the United States every two years, as required by law.[4] Some are seen every three or four years. That's a lot of time between inspections.

Even more alarming is what the FDA doesn't do abroad. Not long ago, most of the medicines used in the United States were made domestically. Over the last decade or so, more and more of our drugs (both prescription and over-the-counter) are made in foreign countries.[5] How do you think big-box discount drugstores are able to charge $4 for a month's supply of fluoxetine when the brand-name Prozac costs over $200? According to the commissioner of the FDA, Margaret Hamburg, MD, "Up to 40 percent of the drugs Americans take are imported, and up to 80 percent of the active pharmaceutical ingredients in those drugs come from foreign sources."[6]

Blind Faith

We would probably be okay with foreign-made pharmaceuticals if the FDA followed the advice Ronald Reagan gave in his farewell address in January 1989. President Reagan cautioned: "It's still trust but verify. It's still play, but cut the cards. It's still watch closely. And don't be afraid to see what you see." The trouble is that the FDA can't watch closely if it is not even looking. About the time we were starting to get messages from readers that they were having problems with generic drugs (1998), the Government Accountability Office (GAO) reported on weaknesses in FDA's foreign inspection program.[7] Over the intervening years, the problems have only gotten worse.[8]

In 2009, the FDA knew of about 3,765 foreign manufacturing plants making drugs for export to the United States from over one hundred different countries.[9] That year, the FDA carried out 424 inspections, or 11 percent of the total. At the rate it's going, it would take the FDA almost a decade to visit every one of the foreign manufacturing plants (that it knows about) just once. Equally alarming, the GAO estimates that 2,394 foreign plants (64 percent) may never have been inspected even *once* by the FDA, including 88 percent of Chinese facilities and 64 percent of Indian manufacturing plants.[10] And in China, the inspectors may often have to let the chemical companies know in advance that an inspection is planned, allowing the facility time to clean up its act.

Self-Policing

"Inspections commonly find unsterile work areas or substandard manufacturing practices, former FDA officials say. Yet the agency relies on paperwork from the plants themselves to determine whether problems have been solved, says Bryan A. Liang, M.D., executive director of the Institute of Health Law Studies at California Western School of Law in San Diego. In many cases, companies can give themselves a clean bill of health. 'The FDA does an inspection and rarely goes back,' Dr. Liang says. 'Anything can happen beyond that point. It's a huge regulatory gap.' "[11]

No other industry so critical to human health is given such slipshod supervision. Airplanes, elevators, and even restaurants are inspected on a regular basis. The majority of the plants overseas where most of the pills are actually made have never been scrutinized. The highly competitive nature of the generic drug market makes low-cost source materials very attractive. Without constant quality surveillance, we worry that manufacturing shortcuts are being taken. Sometimes we even hear from drug company insiders who reinforce our fears.

Spilling the Beans

"I once worked for a pharmaceutical company that ordered a raw ingredient from China. That ingredient was diphenhydramine [an antihistamine found in allergy medicine and many over-the-counter sleeping pills]. I was a quality assurance inspector and had to inspect incoming material. That ingredient was so trashy with what looked like a lot of floor sweepings—black blobs of something I could not identify—that I placed the ingredient on reject. The next day, the boss told me that he had authorized the release of that ingredient to be used in production!

"When I left work later that day, I called the FDA and reported the whole thing. I don't know if the FDA acted on my complaint, but I called in the next day and quit my job."

C. C., April 22, 2009

We assumed that many of the reports of generic problems we were receiving in the mail or seeing on our website were due to lax oversight by the FDA, either in the United States or abroad. On July 10, 2007, China took a drastic step, executing Zheng Xiaoyu, the former head of the Chinese drug regulatory agency, for taking bribes to approve untested and substandard medicine. Zheng started running the Chinese Food and Drug Administration in 1998, around the time we started hearing complaints from consumers.

Zheng's execution didn't end the problem, though. In March 2008, the FDA recalled large quantities of the blood thinner heparin. It turned out that tainted Chinese heparin made from pig intestines was directly linked to over eighty deaths in the United States. Chondroitin sulfate had been added to the heparin to stretch supplies and boost income.

Despite all the headlines and hand wringing over the heparin disaster, Chinese regulatory authorities never cooperated fully with the FDA to investigate the problem or reveal what went wrong.[12]

Chinese drug manufacturers aren't the only ones suspected of taking shortcuts. Ranbaxy was one of India's largest drug companies and one of the top-ten generic drug manufacturers in the world. It supplied large numbers of generics to the U.S. market. In 2005, a whistle-blower inside the company warned about altered test data and raw materials obtained from unapproved sources. In 2008, investigators accused Ranbaxy of falsifying statements and fabricating information about its drugs. U.S. prosecutors alleged that the company forged documents regarding drug quality and covered up violations of manufacturing practices. There were also accusations that the company failed to report patient complaints about certain drugs, such as fluoxetine (the generic form of Prozac), in a timely manner. In September 2008, the FDA finally issued an import alert that effectively banned Ranbaxy from selling thirty different drugs in the U.S. market.

Lest you think all the generic drug manufacturing problems occur only in countries like India and China, one need look no farther than Falls River, New Jersey. According to the nonprofit Institute for Safe Medication Practices, "More than 1000 patient deaths have now been reported in connection with the recall of 800 million digoxin tablets manufactured in New Jersey by the Actavis Group [an Icelandic drug company]. The tablets were recalled because of the possibility that the strength of tablets was greater than labeled and might provide a potentially lethal overdose to patients taking the drug to aid failing hearts. . . . Furthermore, a new recall of digoxin tablets in March 2009 from another manufacturer—Caraco Pharmaceutical Laboratories [owned by Sun Pharmaceutical of India]—underlines weaknesses in the U.S. system for insuring quality control in the manufacture of generic drugs."[13]

A perspective in the New England Journal of Medicine in August 2009 alerted physicians to potential problems with generic drugs.[14] A case was described in which a person had overcome his irregular heart rhythm (atrial fibrillation) from 2001 until 2008 while taking the brand-name beta blocker Toprol XL. When he was switched to generic metoprolol ER made by the Ethex Corporation, this patient developed congestion, breathlessness, and an irregular heart rhythm. The patient reported this problem to the FDA. " 'The only change in my life was the change to the generic,' he said. When he complained to the Food and Drug Administration (FDA), he 'received a reply that all generics are the same.' "[15] Here's the rest of the story: several months after his heart rhythm problem was diagnosed, "Ethex recalled its long-acting metoprolol along with dozens of other generic medicines after the FDA cited more than 35 manufacturing deficiencies at its St. Louis plant."[16]

Fundamental Flaws at the FDA

Until February 2007, we assumed that most of the complaints we were receiving about generic drugs had to do with manufacturing problems in the supply chain. We concluded that the FDA's lax oversight at home and abroad was allowing unscrupulous drugmakers to scam the system with some poor-quality products that somehow managed to make it into the U.S. distribution system. We never imagined that the FDA's generic drug approval process might also have flaws.

The first inkling of something strange came to our e-mail inbox on February 25, 2007, from J. in Dansville, New York. She wrote: "I have been taking Budeprion XL 300 mg for three months instead of Wellbutrin XL 300 mg. I find that I am easily upset and cry very easily. Sometimes I feel aggressive. I also have short, stabbing pains in my head. Taking the brand-name drug (Wellbutrin) helped me feel the best I have felt in twenty years—not depressed and able to enjoy being with my family and friends." That e-mail and the dozens of similar messages that followed over the next several weeks took us into an Alice-in-Wonderland world of generic drug woe and intrigue.

Wellbutrin XL 300 is a long-acting antidepressant that is quite different from Prozac (fluoxetine), Paxil (paroxetine), Zoloft (sertraline), and all other antidepressants on the market. Instead of affecting the neurotransmitter serotonin, Wellbutrin, known generically as bupropion, works in part by modifying a chemical in the brain called dopamine. Unlike SSRI-type drugs, Wellbutrin is far less likely to cause sexual side effects and some of the other classic complications linked to Prozac-like pills.

The original Wellbutrin was approved by the FDA on December 30, 1985. It would have been the first of a new wave of antidepressants preceding Prozac, which wasn't given the green light by the FDA until two years later. Before Wellbutrin could actually hit pharmacy shelves in 1986, however, the FDA called it back. A report of seizures at doses between 400 and 600 mg delayed marketing until 1989. By then, Prozac had taken the market by storm. The original formulation of Wellbutrin also suffered from a significant disadvantage: it had to be taken three times a day because it was very short acting. Most people preferred to take a once-daily pill like Prozac or Paxil.

A longer-acting version of Wellbutrin (SR for "sustained release") was approved in 1996. It was an improvement over the immediate release pill, as it had to be taken only twice daily, but it still lacked the convenience of drugs like Prozac. Finally, in 2003, the FDA approved a more patient-friendly formulation called Wellbutrin XL (XL for "extended release") that needed to be swallowed only once a day. This may all seem like way too much detail, but it unlocks a little-recognized problem in generic drug development and a vulnerability in the FDA's approval process and determination of bioequivalence.

Most physicians, pharmacists, and patients assume that all a drug manufacturer needs to do to get approval from the FDA to market a generic version of a brand-name medicine is duplicate the original pill. Then the company must prove the medicine gets into the bloodstream in a similar or "bioequivalent" manner to the brand name. That is a fallacy. Although the innovator drug loses a patent on the active ingredient in its pill, the actual formulation or delivery system often remains under patent and cannot be copied. This is especially true for many long-acting or extended-release formulations. As a result, the generic company may have to come up with a different process to release the active drug. The company (Biovail) that developed the extended-release formulation for Wellbutrin XL used what is called a membrane technology. When the drug lost its patent, the long-acting delivery system was still protected. The generic manufacturers had to come up with a completely different way to get the active ingredient bupropion into the bloodstream.

Generic Grief

"I have been having problems with Budeprion (generic Wellbutrin) ever since my insurance company changed the prescription over from brand name to generic. Some of the symptoms I've experienced include dizziness, nausea, sleep problems, headaches, body aches, extreme irritability, loss of sex drive, digestive problems, and continuous break-through bleeding. I've been on it for six weeks. I've experienced these side effects ever since the first time I've taken it."

K. Trevor, March 27, 2007

Teva Pharmaceutical Industries is the largest generic drugmaker in the world. In 2006, the FDA approved a generic version of Wellbutrin XL 300 that was manufactured by Impax Laboratories and distributed by Teva under the name Budeprion XL 300. Instead of using a membrane technology, the generic formulation relied on what is called an erodible matrix system. This is a completely different way to release the active drug. Wellbutrin XL 300 was a small round tablet, whereas the generic Budeprion XL 300 was a much larger oval pill. The generic Budeprion XL 300 started showing up on pharmacy shelves in December 2006. By February, we were starting to hear complaints.

At first, we were suspicious. So many people were complaining of similar problems that we considered the possibility that this was a campaign created by the brand-name company GlaxoSmithKling (GSK) to discredit the generic drug. These were patients who said they had taken Wellbutrin XL 300 successfully for years without problems. Within weeks of being switched to the generic formulation, they were reporting symptoms such as headache, anxiety, irritability, nausea, dizziness, insomnia, tremor, mood swings, and panic attacks. Many said that their depression had returned or gotten much worse, and some said they became suicidal, something they maintained had never occurred before.

The stories were coming from all over the country, and they were different enough that we began to believe something strange was happening. On April 16, 2007, we included the following story in our syndicated newspaper column: "I have taken Wellbutrin XL for two years, and it has taken care of my depression beautifully. In January, my insurance company switched me to the generic called Budeprion XL. I didn't think twice about it. I just assumed it was as good as Wellbutrin XL. After a few months thinking I was losing my mind and that Wellbutrin just wasn't working anymore, it finally dawned on me that I was no longer taking *Wellbutrin!* (I honestly hadn't even thought about the generic.) I have been very depressed, crying, and irritable, with no energy or ambition. While I am not suicidal, it sure doesn't sound like a bad plan most days. I will stop Budeprion XL immediately even though I will have to pay full price for Wellbutrin XL."

That story opened the floodgates. First dozens and then hundreds of people sent or e-mailed us stories about suffering side effects and therapeutic failure on the generic. They were so powerful that we could not stand idly by. We forwarded many of these messages on to the highest levels of the FDA but received virtually nothing back in the way of answers. The FDA's position seemed to boil down to "it's all in their heads." The agency maintained that people with depression have ups and downs. If they experience symptoms after switching to Budeprion XL 300, it's pure coincidence. If they got better when going back to the brand-name Wellbutrin XL 300, it was more coincidence. The FDA's explanation was unsatisfying, to say the least.

Budeprion Problems

"I just had a nightmare experience switching from brand-name Wellbutrin 300 mg to the generic "Wellbutrin" called Budeprion 300 mg. I wanted to add my voice to a long list of others.

"I have no history of suicidality, but a day after switching to the generic, I went into a week of steadily rising panic. Then I hit rock bottom this last Saturday. Like some demon took over my body. I wanted to die, felt like someone was holding me by the throat and pressing me against the wall. I was psychotic, self-loathing way, *way* beyond anything I have ever experienced.

"I made it through the worst of it, called a suicide hotline, took two Ativan, and didn't take any more of the Budeprion. The next day, I felt much better and today I'm back to my normal self.

"The pharmacists and the drug companies are adamant that the generics are *the same*. This is, I believe, wrong, and dangerously so."

F. G., May 25, 2007

We contacted Tod Cooperman, MD, president of ConsumerLab .com, a company that tests dietary supplements, herbs, and vitamins, and asked him to check on the purity and safety of this formulation. Dr. Cooperman arranged for dissolution testing: in other words, how rapidly does the pill release its active ingredients in a simulated stomach environment? To our amazement, the generic Budeprion XL 300 performed quite differently than the brand name Wellbutrin XL 300.

In the dissolution tests, GSK's Wellbutrin XL 300 released 8 percent of its active ingredient after two hours, while Teva's Budeprion XL 300 released 34 percent (more than four times as much). After four hours, Wellbutrin XL 300 had released 25 percent, whereas Budeprion XL 300 had released 49 percent.[17-18] This might explain why so many people were complaining about classic symptoms of too much bupropion—headache, nausea, tremor, agitation, anxiety, and irritability. It might also explain why the antidepressant benefits were disappearing. High levels in the morning and lower levels of active drug later in the day might create a roller-coaster effect in the brain.

Perhaps because of our constant badgering or because the FDA was feeling pressure from the media, the agency eventually released the bioequivalence test results between Budeprion XL 300 and Wellbutrin XL 300.[19] These are the data about actual blood levels in human subjects. The first thing we noticed was that the key study was conducted with 150 mg pills, half of the dose that was actually approved. In other words, the FDA *never* required the generic manufacturer to conduct a study on Budeprion XL 300, the product it approved for sale in December 2006. This is irregular.

Imagine going to an eye doctor for your annual exam and having her write a prescription for new glasses based solely on a test of your right eye. No ophthalmologist would ever take such a leap of faith, and yet the FDA took a huge leap of faith when it approved a 300 mg formulation based on data from a 150 mg pill. We suspect that most physicians, pharmacists, and patients do not realize the FDA sometimes approves drugs for which it has not required actual test results.

The second thing we discovered was that the human data paralleled the dissolution data. The generic formula reached its maximum blood concentrations in two to three hours, compared to five or six hours for Wellbutrin, but the FDA said those differences "were not considered clinically significant."[20]

The pieces to the puzzle all seemed to come together. First dozens, then scores and eventually hundreds and hundreds of patients contacted us to relate the problems they were having with this generic antidepressant. Their stories, while different in detail, all seemed to boil down to (1) they experienced a range of symptoms consistent with too much drug in their systems too fast and (2) a loss of antidepressant effect. Then we learned that the formulation technology differed dramatically between the two drugs. Dissolution data demonstrated that the brand name released its active ingredient bupropion more gradually than the generic formulation Budeprion. When the FDA finally published its data on blood levels, it confirmed that indeed the pills performed differently in humans.

Sandy Walsh, a spokeswoman for the FDA, responded to a journalist's question in 2008 about possible generic problems: "If we see scientific evidence that a product is not performing as expected, we will take action. The FDA cannot offer examples where generics have not performed as expected because there have been none for the agency to report."[21] In other words, like the three monkeys: "See no evil, hear no evil, speak no evil."

Veteran's Dilemma

"I'm a disabled veteran and was prescribed Wellbutrin by a Veterans Affairs (VA) doctor. When the VA pharmacy switched to generic Budeprion, I felt the difference *immediately*.

"I woke up thinking that it would just be easier if I died. I have *never, ever* had these kinds of thoughts before, so I saw my doctor the same day. She told me that the FDA only requires a generic drug to have 80 percent of the same quantity as the brand name for approval.

"I am still recuperating from a combat-related injury and have no other insurance, so my family is helping me pay out-of-pocket for brand-name Wellbutrin.

"Please help me get the word out to the FDA and our representatives in Congress *before* someone gets hurt or even commits suicide because of the generic. Go to FDA.gov and fill out an application to report this bad drug! I've even written to Oprah! Maybe we can get insurance companies to recognize the difference, and fewer of us will be paying out-of-pocket."

Navy veteran, November 5, 2010

To this day, we continue to receive heartbreaking stories from people who insist that one or another generic formula of Wellbutrin XL 300 does not work well for them. We now have grave doubts about the

FDA's approval process. If there are problems with generic Wellbutrin, there could be problems with dozens of other medications. For years, the agency's official stance has been that generic drugs are "identical" to their brand-name counterparts. This has allowed insurance companies, hospitals, nursing homes, and discount drugstores to purchase the cheapest generic drugs they could find from whatever source is available. If someone complained, all an insurance company had to do was quote the FDA's mantra that all generic drugs are exactly the same as brand-name drugs. Any perceived problems must be due to the patient's imagination. We think we have demonstrated beyond a reasonable doubt that not all generic drugs are "identical" to their brand-name counterparts.

Generic Epilepsy Medicine

"I took Keppra for epilepsy. In January 2009, I was given generic Keppra (levetiracetam). I felt sick to my stomach and had multiple seizures. My neurologist told me to stay on the brand med and even wrote 'brand necessary' on the script, but the insurance company refused and gave me the generic.

"I had seizures for five weeks before they allowed me to go back on the brand name. My blood level on the generic was much lower than on the brand name, and I found the generic was not as effective."

M. D., March 15, 2009

Within a couple of years it is likely that generic drugs will control 85 percent of the pharmaceutical marketplace.[22] Without better FDA oversight, we fear there could be a train wreck ahead. There is a glimmer of hope, though. Janet Woodcock, MD, is director of the FDA's Center for Drug Evaluation and Research. She is one of the most important leaders at the agency. On October 20, 2010, she gave a speech to the Generic Pharmaceutical Association. For the first time, an FDA official publicly stated that "I've heard it enough times from enough people to believe that there are a few products that aren't meeting quality standards. They say, 'I know there are products out there that aren't equivalent,' and typically they're manufacturing folks."[23]

In other words, employees (industry insiders) have whispered in Dr. Woodcock's ear about their own concerns regarding quality control. In her speech, she also suggested that the FDA may tighten standards in its generic drug approval process. Other countries, like Australia, Japan, Canada, and the European Union, have stricter standards for "critical dose drugs" such as the blood thinner warfarin (Coumadin), the heart drug digoxin (Lanoxin), the antiseizure medicine phenytoin (Dilantin), and lithium, a drug used to treat manic depression (bipolar disorder). We feel vindicated that such a high-placed FDA official now admits that there could be improvements in the FDA's oversight of generic drugs.

Top 10 Tips for Taking Generic Drugs

Until the FDA gets its house in order and has the resources to monitor all domestic and foreign manufacturing plants every two years (as called for by law), we think patients, pharmacists, nurses, and physicians need to be extra vigilant. We cannot assume that all generic drugs are perfect. In fact, we cannot even assume that all brand-name drugs are perfect. Johnson and Johnson is a huge brand-name pharmaceutical company (producer of Tylenol) that got itself into terrible trouble because of manufacturing problems at plants in Puerto Rico and in Fort Washington and Lancaster, Pennsylvania. GlaskoSmithKline, another huge drug company (producer of Paxil), had to pay a fine of $750 million in 2010 because of contaminated drugs it knowingly sold to Medicare and Medicaid patients.[24] If giant brand-name companies that are inspected regularly by the FDA can turn out tainted drugs, how much confidence can we have that small generic manufacturing plants in China or India that have *never* been inspected are performing to accepted standards?

Given the flaws in the FDA's system for generic drug approval and oversight, we have come up with some suggestions for consumers and health professionals so that generic drugs can be used in a safer manner. Although our recommendations are not foolproof, they offer some guidance for saving money on medicine without putting your life at risk.

1. **Make no assumptions.** It would be a mistake to assume that your generic drug is flawed, just as it would be a mistake to assume it is perfect. You will need to assess the effectiveness of your medicine.

2. **Keep track of the manufacturer.** Ask the pharmacist to always put the name of the generic manufacturer on your prescription bottle. There may be dozens of different companies making your medicine. You will need to keep track of which ones make the pills that work for you.

3. **Keep records.** Objective measurements such as blood sugar and blood pressure will allow you to track progress. If your numbers are under control, your medicine is likely working. If they change after a substitution, you may need to revert to the brand name or a different generic manufacturer.

4. **Ask for your lab results.** Your physician should supply you with all lab results so you can plot any changes. That includes blood lipids (fats) such as total cholesterol, LDL (low-density lipoprotein) and HDL (high-density lipoprotein) cholesterol, and triglycerides. If you are on a blood thinner such as warfarin (Coumadin), you will want your INR (international normalized ratio) values or PT (prothrombin) numbers. If you have diabetes, the HbA1c is an important value to follow. Should

your numbers change dramatically after a drug substitution, let your doctor know *immediately.*

5. **Monitor symptoms.** There are conditions that aren't measured in numbers but that can be objectively evaluated. An antiseizure medicine can be assumed to be working if you don't have a seizure. On the other hand, seizures are a strong indication that a generic drug isn't doing its job. Likewise, a medication that is supposed to alleviate urinary symptoms for a man with prostate problems can be judged by how many times the gentleman has to get up to pee at night.

6. **Listen to your body.** Some important health problems are subjective. Pain and mood can't be measured with a test, but you know how you feel. Write it down in a diary. If your pain comes roaring back after switching to a generic pain reliever, perhaps the medication has a problem. Based on what you have read earlier in this chapter, you know that problems after switching to a generic can also happen with depression.

7. **Challenge and rechallenge.** This is a time-honored way to assess a person's reaction to medication. If generic drug X causes a headache, going back on the brand name should solve the problem. To confirm that the difficulty lies with the generic, taking it again to see if the symptom reappears is the rechallenge.

8. **Be assertive.** If your physician or pharmacist insists that all generic drugs are identical to their brand-name counterparts, ask them to read this chapter. Now that Dr. Woodcock, one of the FDA's leading administrators, has herself admitted that she has heard of problems, your physician and pharmacist may be more willing to consider the possibility of differences among formulations.

9. **Seek allies.** Ask your physician and pharmacist to go to bat for you if your insurance company balks at paying for the brand name. If you

find a generic drug from a particular manufacturer works, stick with it, and make sure your pharmacy keeps it on hand or orders it just for you.

10. Report any problems to the Food and Drug Administration. The only way the FDA can investigate a potential problem is by starting with a MedWatch report. You will find the form online at www.fda.gov/medwatch. There is also a phone number: 1-800-332-1088.

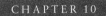

CHAPTER 10

THE SCREWING OF SENIOR CITIZENS

Americans are living longer than ever before, but many are enjoying their extra years less and less. That is caused in part by medicines that are supposed to help but end up hurting instead. People aged sixty-five and older currently make up 12.6 percent of the population, though that percentage will soon rise dramatically.[1] Senior citizens take one-third of all the prescription medications.[2-4] Seniors living independently in the community take an extraordinary number of pills. According to one survey, roughly 40 percent take five different drugs a week, and 12 percent take ten or more medications.[5] People taking seven or more meds simultaneously have an 82 percent chance of experiencing an adverse drug reaction.[6] Too many of the multiple medicines seniors swallow are prescribed inappropriately and lead to serious side effects, hospitalization, and death.[7]

Seniors with multiple medical problems are also more likely to be hospitalized, and while they are in the hospital, they may be at particular risk. The Department of Health and Human Services examined this issue, and the report issued by the Inspector General in 2010 is chilling.[8] The researchers analyzed the medical records of 780 Medicare patients hospitalized during October 2008. Approximately one out of four suffered harm from their hospital care. The investigators estimated that 15,000 Medicare recipients died each month as a result of care they received in the hospital. That means an annual death toll of almost 200,000 senior citizens precipitated by adverse events experienced in hospitals. According to the Inspector General, nearly half the problems were avoidable.

The stories come in like the tide. A mother used to play golf, attend social gatherings, and keep up with grandchildren. But gradually she finds it difficult to walk and swing a golf club and loses interest in friends and family. No one thinks to associate her insidious decline with the various drugs she is taking. Instead, more medicine is added to aid with insomnia, anxiety, and depression. The decline accelerates, and family members conclude age has finally caught up with her.

Drug-Induced Depression

"My eighty-six-year-old father was hospitalized a year ago for a stomach bug—high fever and vomiting—an eight-hour drive from where I live. Within two months, he had been sent to four different hospitals and two rehab units. The last hospital was a locked-down geriatric psychiatric hospital because he was in acute psychosis due to the medications he had been put on. I had to move him to where I live so that I could take over his care.

"He's now almost back to normal, although there are some lasting results. He had been a vibrant part of the community, driving and sitting on two local boards until this happened. My parents' lives were turned upside down.

"I requested copies of all his records from all the facilities, and it was unbelievable how many misdiagnoses there were. Most of his problems had been caused by new medications that they put him on—side effects and drug interactions. The doctors are on their rounds so early that you have to ambush them at 6:00 in the morning to talk to them. *Do it!* Make friends with the nurses. They can be your allies."

We are deluged with messages from people worried about older relatives. One woman wrote: "My husband and I are concerned about his eighty-one-year-old father. He has almost no energy, is short of breath, and has digestive problems. His medications include: Nitrobid for his heart, Zantac for digestion, verapamil and aspirin for heart, lovastatin for cholesterol, prednisone for polymyalgia rheumatica, naproxen for joints, furosemide for excess fluid, Nasonex for allergies, meclizine for dizziness, calcium for bones, Detrol and Flomax for his bladder. Is he taking too many medications?"

Dizziness, drowsiness, and digestive problems are common side effects from some of the dozen drugs this man is taking. Trying to treat adverse drug reactions with more medicine is like trying to get out of debt by borrowing more money. It is a never-ending downward spiral. Drug-induced dizziness and drowsiness can easily lead to a fall that can lead to a broken hip. When an older person breaks a bone, it can be as lethal as many cancers.[9]

Paying a High Price for Pills

The following author conclusions were based on a study of more than 30,000 Medicare patients aged sixty-five years or older participating in a New England–based multispecialty group practice:

"If the findings of the present study are generalized to the population of all Medicare enrollees, then more than 1,900,000 adverse drug events—more than a quarter of which are preventable—occur each year among 38 million Medicare enrollees; furthermore, estimates based on our study suggest that there are in excess of 180,000 life-threatening or fatal adverse drug events per year, of which more than 50 percent may be preventable."[10]

P.S.: "These estimates are likely to be conservative." In other words, the actual problem is likely far worse.

We are not revealing a deep, dark secret. Experts have known for decades that senior citizens are being prescribed way too many dangerous drugs. A CDC (Centers for Disease Control and Prevention) researcher estimated that inappropriate medications were prescribed at as many as 16.7 million doctor visits in the year 2000.[11] The investigators who understand the scope of the problem keep begging for change, but their pleas have fallen on deaf ears. Inappropriate prescribing for the elderly is so common today, it is almost taken for granted. Most doctors are just not trained adequately about the special needs of senior citizens. In one study of physician knowledge about prescribing to elderly patients, 71 percent scored poorly. Despite their bad showing,

75 percent of those surveyed felt confident prescribing drugs to older people.[12]

Mismedication of the Elderly

In 1989, the Inspector General of the United States, Richard Kusserow, issued a report called *Medicare Drug Utilization Review*. The results were horrifying, but nothing has been done over the intervening years to change the situation. If anything, the problem has gotten substantially worse.

- 200,000 older Americans were hospitalized in 1987 because of adverse reactions to their medicines or because they developed a bad reaction while in the hospital.
- 63,000 senior citizens experienced mental impairment annually that was either brought on by or exacerbated by medication.
- 32,000 older people broke a hip every year because a medicine led to a fall.[13]

A Scarcity of Specialists

According to the American Academy of Pediatrics, there are over 80,000 pediatricians and pediatric specialists practicing in the United States.[14] They take care of 60 million children. By contrast, there are only about 7,000 geriatricians (doctors who specialize in caring for older patients), and their numbers have been declining.[15] By 2020 there will be over 50 million senior citizens, but that is just the tip of the iceberg. With 78 million baby boomers headed for retirement, it won't be long before there are more senior citizens than young people. There will not be anywhere close to enough knowledgeable physicians or related health care providers to care for them. It is one of the scariest, most shameful screwups in medicine!

Don't take our word for it. The Institute of Medicine (IOM) is arguably the most prestigious, unbiased, and authoritative organization making health policy recommendations in America. A committee of the IOM released a report in 2008 that let the cat out of the bag.[16] John Rowe, MD, is one of the country's most prominent geriatricians. He was the founding director of the Division on Aging at the Harvard Medical School and chaired the IOM committee. In testimony to the U.S. Senate, Dr. Rowe revealed a "looming crisis that is quickly approaching: the considerable shortfall in the quality and organization of the health care workforce to care for tomorrow's older Americans."[17]

Dr. John Rowe on the Future of Geriatric Care

"How adequate is our health care workforce supply to meet these impending needs?

"The answer is quite simple: we are woefully unprepared. The U.S. health care system is in denial about the impending demands. Little has been done to prepare the health care workforce for the aging of our nation and the current supply and organization of the health care workforce will simply be inadequate to meet the needs of the older adults of the future."[18]

The future is now. We are already experiencing a huge shortfall in experienced professionals capable of handling the special needs of aging baby boomers and their parents. Even though many experts have been warning that this day was coming, there are no quick fixes for this crisis.

So how did it happen? Blame modern medicine and a hierarchical culture that medical educators have fostered for decades. Geriatrics is not sexy. Medical students are not encouraged to consider going into this field. If anything, they are discouraged. A perfect example is the story of Amit Shah, MD. After medical school, Dr. Shah opted for a geriatrics fellowship at Johns Hopkins University. He quickly discovered that other doctors looked down on him for this choice. The most discouraging reaction was from a pulmonologist during Dr. Shah's residency. "When I passed him in the hall, he would shake his head and mutter, 'Waste of a mind,' " he said. "My retort was always that the geriatric population is often the most complicated, not only medically but also socially and psychologically, and that was exactly the specialization you should want your top students going into." [19]

Most medical schools in the United States do not have departments of geriatrics the way they have departments of pediatrics, dermatology, or neurology. Students are rarely required to take course work in geriatric medicine.[20] Because mentors talk up specialties such as cardiology, surgery, or orthopedics and ignore geriatrics, it is hardly any wonder that few students consider a career taking care of "geezers" and "gomers," (an acronym doctors coined for "get out of my emergency room"). Although the typical U.S. physician will prescribe huge numbers of medications to older people, the chances are overwhelming that the doctor will never have received adequate training in how to do so properly.[21]

Turning Away a "Gomer"

When Joe's uncle Leo had a recurrence of his prostate cancer, he was prescribed DES (diethylstilbestrol, a potent estrogen) to control symptoms and slow the spread of the disease. Several months after starting on DES, he developed chest pain. This energetic eighty-four-year-old retired dairy farmer had trouble catching his breath, and walking up stairs became difficult.

His doctors twice disregarded his discomfort, not taking into consideration the fact that Leo wasn't a complainer. When the stabbing pain in his chest got so severe he couldn't stand it anymore, he decided he had best take himself to the local emergency department at a top-notch teaching hospital.

The doctors there didn't take him seriously, either. He was sent home with a pain reliever even after he suggested it could be a blood clot in his lungs caused by the medicine he was taking (a well-known side effect of DES). It took precious weeks before his physicians finally figured out that Leo was indeed suffering from a pulmonary embolism that could easily have been fatal.

If you want further proof of the low esteem medicine holds for geriatricians, just follow the money. Cardiologists, radiologists, and orthopedic surgeons can all expect to make more than $400,000 annually. Physicians who specialize in older people, however, are at the bottom of the medical income ladder, often earning less than a general internist.[22] It doesn't take a medical student or a resident long to figure out that specializing in geriatric medicine is not valued either by most of their instructors or society as a whole. Contrast this dismal situation with Great Britain, where every medical school has a department of geriatric medicine and physicians are compensated better for treating senior citizens. Guess what: geriatrics is the third most popular specialty in the United Kingdom.[23]

Why It Matters!

You might be asking yourself whether this is all much ado about nothing. What's the big deal about geriatricians anyway? Why can't older people see a family practice physician or an internist like everyone else? Just as pediatricians know that children are not mini-adults and often require specialized treatments, geriatricians understand that dosing requirements and physiology often differ for someone who is seventy-something compared with someone who is thirty-something. Kidney and liver function change with age and require careful assessment so drug doses can be calculated correctly. Older brains may be much more susceptible to drug side effects than younger brains. The antihistamine diphenhydramine (DPH) in drugs like Tylenol PM, Excedrin PM, and Nytol, for example, can be quite sedating. A twenty-four-year-old may handle it reasonably well when the drug is swallowed at bedtime. An eighty-four-year-old might be more vulnerable to DPH-induced side effects such as unsteadiness, especially if she had to get up in the middle of the night to pee. A fall could be catastrophic.

Senior citizens frequently have chronic conditions such as high blood pressure, arthritis, breathing problems, or heart trouble. Such health problems are rarely cured. They have to be managed, and that requires listening, patience, empathy, counseling, and compassion. Most important of all, there must be coordination of care. A busy internist who is terrific at treating diseases in middle-aged patients may become frustrated and impatient with a frail elderly person who moves and talks slowly, complains about drug side effects, and sees a variety of specialists who prescribe multiple medications and offer contradictory advice.

"Dysorganized" Care

"Despite increasing recognition of the need for integrated, comprehensive, patient-centered primary care as the focal point for health care delivery, especially in older patients, the recent US health care legislation did little to foster the adoption of such a model, leaving the existing fragmented, overspecialized system of care generally intact. Such 'dysorganization' is particularly problematic for complex patients with several chronic conditions who take multiple medications, often provided by numerous specialists in little or no contact with one another—a recipe for pharmacological chaos."[24]

Jerry Avorn, MD, Harvard Medical School, in *JAMA*, October 13, 2010

This is why geriatricians are the last line of defense for older people. They are one-third less likely to prescribe inappropriate medications than other physicians.[25] Geriatric experts can also coordinate care administered by multiple specialists. When they see a medical colleague treating the numbers rather than the whole patient, they can intervene. Take cholesterol, for example. Everyone knows that elevated cholesterol levels are a risk factor for heart disease in middle-aged men. A cardiologist or an internist might do a routine blood test in an older woman and discover elevated cholesterol. The reflex is often to dash off a prescription for Crestor, Lipitor, or some other statin-type cholesterol-lowering drug. In Sweden, roughly one-third of those aged seventy-five to eighty-four are given statins.[26] It is safe to assume that older people in the United States are also being prescribed statins at a comparable rate.

There is only one problem with this program. There are no good data demonstrating that lowering cholesterol in senior citizens, especially those over eighty, saves lives.[27] There is even the possibility that giving statins to older people who don't have heart disease might shorten their lives.[28] Studies suggest that older people with total cholesterol levels below 212 appear to be at higher risk for death than those with higher levels. Those with total cholesterol levels around 230 actually live longest.[29] Low LDL (low-density lipoprotein) cholesterol levels have been linked to a higher risk of bleeding stroke and Parkinson's disease.[30-31] Also worrisome are studies that note an association between low total and LDL cholesterol levels and an increased incidence of cancer.[32-34] (We must note that the cancer connection is highly controversial and remains one of those chicken-or-egg questions. In other words, doctors aren't sure whether undiagnosed cancer lowers cholesterol or whether low cholesterol contributes to the development of cancer.)

Regardless, no data show that lowering cholesterol in otherwise healthy seniors will prolong their lives, and there is a lot of evidence of some serious side effects, including muscle pain and weakness and perhaps even cognitive complications. A geriatrician is likely to understand that quality of life is crucial for healthy aging. Such a physician can intercede on behalf of an older person to prevent the "cure" from becoming worse than the disease.

Numbers vs. Quality of Life

"My father started taking simvastatin (Zocor), and within a year, our family started noticing loss of memory. It got worse, and he started getting pain in his legs. Over the next year, he went downhill and was hospitalized for congestive heart failure.

"Our family couldn't figure it out. Before that, he was healthy despite bad eating habits. He still had good muscle tone, was very active, and walked erect, and we had great conversations. My sister and I started asking questions and discovered that his doctor had prescribed the statin to lower his cholesterol about a year before we noticed his change in health.

"We know in our hearts that the drug was responsible. We started researching the side effects of statins ourselves and were shocked to find out we were not the only ones to draw this conclusion. Finally, when Dad went in for open-heart surgery to replace a mitral valve to help with congestive heart failure, we insisted that Dad not go back on the statin. Zocor didn't prevent congestive heart failure.

"My sister and I had to fight his doctors and my mother, who believes doctors are always right. Since then, though, Dad's memory has come back, and he is able to walk much better."

Finding a geriatrician may not be easy. Remember, there is a shortage, and it will only get worse over the next several years. Nevertheless, the American Geriatrics Society is a nonprofit group of health professionals "devoted to improving the health, independence and quality of life of all older people." The website www.americangeriatrics.org has a referral search system that will allow you to find a geriatrics health care provider in many communities. There is also a printed list available by calling 1-800-247-4779.

Doing Your Homework

In the event that you cannot find someone who specializes in geriatric care, you will need to become ever more vigilant and take matters into your own hands for yourself or for an older relative or friend. The first step is locating a primary care provider with some knowledge of geriatric medicine. The only way to find out is to ask your doctor if she has received extra training in this field. Even if you can't find someone with expertise in treating senior citizens, you need someone who at least *likes* caring for older people and is flexible, patient, and compassionate. This person will need to coordinate care with any other specialists you may see and to double-check to make sure all the medications, nutrients, and dietary supplements you take are compatible.

The next step is to become informed and ask lots of questions. Do not assume that your nurse practitioner, family practice physician, internist, pharmacist, or medical specialist understands the special needs of seniors. Whenever a medication is proposed, ask the prescriber if there are any special considerations regarding older patients. The prescribing information that comes with most modern medicines has a special section on geriatric use. It can advise about special dosing adjustments or side effects related to senior citizens. There's one last question, and it's really important. Ask if the medicine is on the Beers List. If the prescriber looks at you with a blank stare, there's a problem.

The Beers Criteria: Beware Bad Drugs

Over twenty years ago, geriatrician Mark Beers, MD, and a team of colleagues from Harvard studied medication use in twelve Massachusetts nursing homes. They tracked 850 patients over the course of one full month. The researchers were dismayed to discover that more than half the residents were receiving either sedatives, sleeping pills, antidepressants, or antipsychotic medications.[35] Many of the prescriptions were for inappropriate drugs that were likely to cause confusion, sedation, and disorientation as well as dry mouth, dizziness, and constipation.

Dr. Beers was so affected by this research that he went on to organize an expert panel that produced a list of medications generally considered inappropriate for elderly patients. It was called the Beers criteria (or Beers List) and was published in 1991.[36] This landmark consensus effort has helped geriatricians determine which medications should probably be avoided, if possible, in senior citizens. The Beers criteria were revised in 2003.[37] Since Dr. Beers's landmark effort, there have been other efforts to help prescribers avoid inappropriate medications for the elderly, such as IPET (Improved Prescribing in the Elderly Tool), the McLeod criteria, and the MAI (Medication Appropriateness Index)

The Beers List[41]
of Drugs Older People Should Generally Avoid

Alprazolam (**Xanax**): *doses greater than 2 mg*

Amiodarone (**Cordarone**)

Amitriptyline (**Elavil**)

Amphetamines and anorexic agents

Barbiturates: *except to control seizures*

Belladonna alkaloids (**Donnatal and others**)

Bisacodyl (**Dulcolax**): *long-term use*

Carisoprodol (**Soma**)

Cascara sagrada: *long-term use*

Chlorazepate (**Tranxene**)

Chlordiazepoxide (**Librium**)

Chlordiazepoxide-amitryptyline (**Limbitrol**)

Chlorpheniramine (**Chlor-Trimeton**)

Chlorpropamide (**Diabinese**)

Chlorzoxazone (**Paraflex**)

Cimetidine (**Tagamet**)

Clidinium-chlordiazepoxide (**Librax**)

Clonodine (**Catapres**)

Cyclandelate (**Cyclospasmol**)

Cyclobenzaprine (**Flexeril**)

Cyproheptadine (**Periactin**)

Desiccated thyroid

Dexchlorpheniramine (**Polaramine**)

Diazepam (**Valium**)

Dicyclomine (**Bentyl**)

Digoxin (**Lanoxin**): *doses greater than 0.125 mg except for atrial arrhythmias*

Diphenhydramine (**Benadryl**)

Dipyridamole (**Persantine**)

Disopyramide (**Norpace and Norpace CR**)

Doxazosin (**Cardura**)

Doxepin (**Sinequan**)

Ergot mesyloids (**Hydergine**)

Estrogens (oral)

Ethacrynic acid (**Edecrin**)

Ferrous sulfate: *doses greater than 325 mg*

Fluoxetine (**Prozac**)

Flurazepam (**Dalmane**)

Guanadrel (**Hylorel**)

Guanethidine (**Ismelin**)

Halazepam (**Paxipam**)

Hydroxyzine (**Atarax, Vistaril**)

Hyoscyamine (**Levsin, Levsinex**)

Indomethacin (**Indocin, Indocin SR**)

Isoxsuprine (**Vasodilan**)

Ketorolac (**Toradol**)

Lorazepam (**Ativan**): *doses greater than 3 mg*

Meperidine (**Demerol**)

Meprobamate (**Equanil, Miltown**)

Mesoridazine (**Serentil**)

Metaxalone (**Skelaxin**)

Methyldopa (**Aldomet**)

Methyldopa-hydrochlorothiazide (**Aldoril**)

Methyltestosterone (**Android, Testrad, Virilon**)

Mineral oil

Naproxen (**Aleve, Avaprox, Naprosyn**): *long-term use*

Neoloid: *long-term use*

Nifedipine (**Adalat, Procardia**)

Nitrofurantoin (**Macrodantin**)

Orphenadrine (**Norflex**)

Oxaprozin (**Daypro**)

Oxazepam (**Serax**): *doses greater than 60 mg*

Oxybutynin (**Ditropan, Ditropan XL**)

Pentazocine (**Talwin**)

Perphenazine-amitriptyline (**Triavil**)

Piroxicam (**Feldene**)

Promethazine (**Phenergan**)

Propantheline (**Pro-Banthine**)

Propoxyphene (**Darvon, Darvon with ASA, Darvon-N, and Darvocet-N**)

Quazepam* (**Doral**)

Reserpine: *doses greater than 3 mg*

Temazepam (**Restoril**): *doses greater than 15 mg*

Thioridazine (**Mellaril**)

Ticlopidine (**Ticlid**)

Triazolam (**Halcion**): *doses greater than 0.25 mg*

Trimethobenzamide (**Tigan**)

Tripelennamine

*Less severe anticholinergic effects

criteria. What is sad, though, is that many primary care providers and nongeriatric specialists have never even heard of the Beers criteria or any of the other tools for avoiding inappropriate prescribing in the elderly. That is why in study after study, roughly one-quarter to one-half of older people end up receiving problem prescriptions.[38-39]

Ignorance of Beers Is Not Bliss for Patients

"From our analysis, it seems that many primary care doctors do not possess a strong understanding and knowledge of PIP [potentially inappropriate prescribing], even though they treat a large number of older patients in multiple care settings.... The majority of doctors were unaware of Beers criteria as a guideline to assist in their prescribing for elderly.... Regardless of their knowledge scores, the majority of doctors are confident with their prescribing in the elderly."[40]

Because there is a strong possibility that your primary care provider will be unfamiliar with the Beers List of generally inappropriate drugs, we are providing the revised list here. Many of these are older medications that are available generically and are therefore less expensive. Beware, though: if side effects lead to serious problems, a bargain medication may be a false economy. However, no one should ever stop medicine without checking with the prescriber. In some cases, these drugs may actually be appropriate for a reason only the prescriber can explain.

Falls and Fractures

When a young or middle-aged person breaks a bone, it hurts like hell and can take several months to heal. When an older person breaks a bone, it can be a life-threatening event, especially if a hip is involved. In the year following a hip fracture, the risk of dying ranges from 14 to 36 percent.[42] Blood clots in the lungs and severe infections are just two of the complications that can end a life prematurely after such an accident. Even when a person survives, there is a strong likelihood there will be substantial time spent in a rehab center or nursing home. Independence and quality of life can be altered permanently. Many senior citizens will be left with chronic pain and disability after such a fracture, and some will never make it out of a nursing home.

Given the horrific consequences of a hip fracture, it is not surprising that physicians are encouraged to do something to prevent this kind of problem. A prescription for a bone-building drug is often their first choice. If you watch any television at all, the chances are good that you have seen commercials for such osteoporosis drugs. Sally Field has told you that Boniva (ibandronate) builds strong, healthy bones to help prevent fractures. Similar bisphosphonate drugs include Actonel (risedronate), Fosamax (alendronate), and Reclast (zoledronic acid). Doctors have been quick to embrace the pharmaceutical solution for fractures. We'll discuss the benefits and risks of these drugs shortly.

When it comes to preventing fractures, however, *avoiding* the kinds of drugs that make you unsteady on your feet may be more important than *taking* drugs that attempt to make bones stronger. That's because over 90 percent of hip fractures are caused by falling.[43] Nearly one-third of people over sixty-five will fall at least once in a year.[44] Falls are responsible for more than four-fifths of the injuries that result in hospitalization and more than two-fifths of admissions to nursing homes. Preventing falls is critical for healthy aging. Unfortunately, many primary care providers may not take this into account when prescribing medications.

There are hundreds of drugs that cause dizziness, drowsiness, and unsteadiness. Some of the worst culprits are antianxiety agents, sedatives, and sleeping pills, which increase the chances for a fall by 50 percent.[45] It is not surprising that benzodiazepine drugs such as Xanax (alprazolam), Klonopin (clonazepam), Valium (diazepam), Dalmane (flurazepam), and Restoril (temezepam) are particularly problematic for older people. They are notorious for causing drowsiness and dizziness as well as impaired coordination and balance.

Most people can understand that sedatives might cause dizziness and imbalance. They may not realize that many blood pressure medications can also cause similar symptoms. An internist who aggressively treats hypertension with multiple medications and leaves a patient dizzy, dazed, and off kilter may dramatically increase the risk for a fall. Even over-the-counter and prescription arthritis drugs and pain relievers (NSAIDs or nonsteroidal anti-inflammatory drugs) can cause dizziness, headaches, and confusion.[46] Given that millions of senior citizens take such medications daily to ease arthritis pain, it comes as a shock to learn that they may also increase the risk for falls.[47]

Aleve and Drowsiness

Q. Can Aleve sometimes cause drowsiness? I only take one, but later I find myself dozing off. Is there a hidden ingredient that causes this? Am I the only one who experiences this problem?

A. Nonsteroidal anti-inflammatory drugs (NSAIDs) such as over-the-counter ibuprofen (Advil, Motrin IB) and naproxen (Aleve) or prescription products like diclofenac (Cataflam, Voltaren), indomethacin (Indocin), and meloxicam (Mobic) can sometimes cause drowsiness, dizziness, or confusion.

You are not the only one who gets sleepy or spacey on medications like Advil or Aleve. A nurse who wrote to us several years ago reported that ibuprofen made her mentally foggy. She feared early onset Alzheimer's disease, but found that stopping the NSAID improved her mental status.

Dizziness, light-headedness, vertigo, or impaired balance are *not* minor side effects. They should be considered extremely dangerous, especially for an older person. Ignoring such symptoms, especially if they are caused by medicine, is a major medical screwup. The prescribing physician must try to find alternatives that do not cause such complications.

Osteoporosis Drugs and Broken Bones

Doctors have enthusiastically embraced medications to prevent or treat osteoporosis. In 2005, nearly 5 million Americans received a prescription for bone drugs like Actonel, Boniva, and Fosamax (available generically as alendronate).[48] These medications are known as bisphosphonates, and they work by slowing the natural breakdown of bone by cells called osteoclasts. This allows bone-building cells (osteoblasts) to catch up a bit and improves bone mineral density. These medications are supposed to prevent fractures. Evidence has been building, however, that these drugs may actually increase the risk of an unusual type of fracture.[49] The Food and Drug Administration (FDA) issued a safety announcement in 2010 warning about atypical fractures of the thigh. These femur fractures can occur without a fall, collision, or trauma. Just walking may bring on this uncommon break.

We had been hearing about these problems long before the FDA issued its warning. One woman reported: "I had been on Fosamax for seven years when I started having leg pain. The doctors I saw could not find anything wrong. Then one morning in the steam room at the gym, my left femur just snapped in half. It was a weird break and I had to have a rod put in. Less than six months later, I was rushing around my son's kitchen getting my grandkids' breakfast, and my right femur broke, making me fall. It broke in the same place as the left, and now I have rods in both legs."

No one yet knows whether the cases of unusual femur fractures are comparable to canaries in the coal mine. They could be a tiny blip on the adverse drug reaction radar screen or the first signs of a potentially huge problem. Remember, it takes years before people start experiencing the early warning signs of trouble (groin or thigh pain that worsens with weight bearing). Experts in bone physiology have pointed out that bisphosphonates can interfere with the natural bone remodeling process that normally helps repair microdamage. This may lead to brittle bones that eventually become vulnerable to fracture.[50]

Fosamax Fiasco

"I took Fosamax for ten years, starting right after it was put on the market. I now have osteonecrosis of the jaw, or ONJ. I have lost two teeth from this and have to be very careful when I have my teeth cleaned to prevent further problems. My dentist cannot figure out what caused my ONJ (I had no tooth extractions or other procedures to trigger it). He had never seen ONJ or had any warnings about it.

"Now they are giving a very brief warning that jaw problems can result from taking Fosamax. Too little, too late for me. I have to be very careful with what happens in my mouth now so as not to lose any more teeth."

As disconcerting as these atypical fractures may be, there are other concerns about bisphosphonates. These osteoporosis drugs are linked to jaw bone death (ONJ, or osteonecrosis of the jaw). They can also cause incapacitating muscle, bone, and joint pain as well as digestive tract irritation. Many physicians are not aware that these drugs can be a source of such debilitating pain. At the time of this writing, the FDA is reviewing data that may link bisphosphonates to a higher risk for esophageal cancer. In addition, an irregular heart rhythm called atrial fibrillation has been associated with injected bisphosphonates given to cancer patients.[51] Whether atrial fibrillation might also occur with oral medicine remains controversial.

Clearly, the final chapter on the benefits of bisphosphonates versus their risks is not in. They may indeed turn out to be wonderful drugs that will dramatically reduce the risk of hip fractures. On the other hand, the potential complications are not trivial. Such drugs should be used only by people who are truly vulnerable to osteoporosis and fractures.

The Dementia Dilemma

There was a time when the "C word" (cancer) was the most dreaded diagnosis you could get. These days the "D word" (dementia) may be even scarier. That's because we have no cure or even good treatments for Alzheimer's disease or any of the other conditions that lead to dementia. Not surprisingly, many older people worry a lot about their failing memories. When they can't match a name to a familiar face or forget a number (PIN, Social Security, phone, password), they joke nervously about a "senior moment." Equally worrisome is cognitive decline—an impairment in judgment, learning, thinking, and comprehension. Words often get scrambled, and people know that they have "slipped" a bit, but they can still function. The underlying fear, though, is that they are on a slippery slope toward Alzheimer's.

Family members, friends, and physicians may assume that Aunt Mabel's cognitive impairment or memory problems are brought on by too many birthdays—in other words, normal aging. What they may not realize is that the problem could be too many drugs, or the wrong type of drugs. There are an amazing number of medications that can throw a monkey wrench into the mental machinery. One of the scariest screwups older people must contend with is their doctor's lack of knowledge about drugs that mess up the mind.

Some of the worst offenders are the anticholinergics. That's a pharmacological term for a class of medications that interfere with the ability of the neurochemical acetylcholine (ACh) to completely bind to nerve cells. ACh is a neurotransmitter that is essential for normal muscle contraction. Every time you lace your shoes, take a step, or type on a computer keyboard acetylcholine is intimately involved in the process. Without this chemical, you couldn't move or breathe. ACh is also essential for memory and proper nervous system function.

Medical students are given a few hours of training about anticholinergic drugs. They are taught about belladonna, extracted from the deadly nightshade plant, and compounds such as atropine and scopolamine. Doctors in training learn that drugs in this class can be used to treat asthma (ipratropium [Atrovent], tiotropium [Spiriva]); motion sickness (scopolamine [Transderm Scop]); diarrhea (atropine plus diphenoxylate [Lomotil], loperamide [Imodium]); irritable bowel syndrome (clidinium plus chlordiazepoxide [Librax], dicyclomine [Bentyl], hyoscyamine [Levsin], methscopolamine [Pamine]); overactive bladder (fesoterodine [Toviaz], oxybutynin [Ditropan], tolteradine [Detrol]); and Parkinson's disease (benztropine [Cogentin], trihexyphenidyl [Artane]). And ophthalmologists are taught that if they want to see the entire eye, they will need to use anticholinergic drops to dilate the pupil.

What physicians may not be taught is that many other drugs also have anticholinergic activity that can cause cognitive dysfunction, memory impairment, impulsive behavior, delirium, and confused thinking, and can increase the risk for falls.[52] Roughly one in five older people takes an anticholinergic medication.[53] When drugs with anticholinergic effects are combined, the risk for problems increases dramatically. Someone who is taking amitryptyline (which is frequently prescribed for nerve pain) along with the diuretic furosemide (Lasix), the heartburn medicine cimetidine (Tagamet), and Tylenol PM (with the antihistamine diphenhydramine) to sleep would be getting a very large anticholinergic load. Side effects could include constipation, dry mouth, blurry vision, and cognitive dysfunction.

The Three-City Study

French researchers tracked 6,912 men and women over four years. None had dementia at the start of the trial. Women taking anticholinergic drugs "showed greater decline over 4 years in verbal fluency scores and in global cognitive functioning than women not using anticholinergic drugs. In men, an association was found with decline in visual memory and to a lesser extent in executive function."

The investigators concluded that "elderly people taking anticholinergic drugs were at increased risk for cognitive decline and dementia. Discontinuing anticholinergic treatments was associated with a decreased risk. Physicians should carefully consider prescription of anticholinergic drugs in elderly people, especially in the very elderly and in persons at high genetic risk for cognitive disorder."[54]

Drugs for overactive bladder can be particularly problematic for older people.[55] They are widely advertised on television, but there is little mention of complications like memory problems or confusion. One reader of our newspaper column described her mother's situation: "My mother was recently prescribed Detrol. She has become increasingly disoriented and has a lot of trouble sleeping. It's really heartbreaking to see her go this way in bits and pieces. She has no appetite or energy, but they keep piling on more and more medication. Her kidney doctor said that Detrol had no side effects, but a regular doctor said it could cause disorientation. Her quality of life (and ours) is suffering. She is becoming less and less able to take care of herself."

The following list of medications does not list every possible drug with anticholinergic activity, but it does include many of the best known. We recognize that some of these medicines may be necessary for certain patients. Heart drugs like digoxin and diuretics such as furosemide, for example, can be essential for patients with congestive heart failure. No one should ever stop any prescription medicine without close medical supervision. Nevertheless, if you or someone you love is taking medicine with anticholinergic effects, please discuss the possible impact on their cognitive function.

Statins and Memory

Anticholinergics aren't the only drugs that can affect memory and cognition. Many doctors have a very hard time believing that statin-type cholesterol-lowering drugs could have an impact on the brain. When

Medications with Anticholinergic Activity[56-57]

Alprazolam (**Xanax**)

Amantadine* (**Symmetrel**)

Amitriptyline (**Elavil**)

Atropine

Baclofen*

Benztropine (**Cogentin**)

Carisoprodol (**Soma**)

Cetirizine* (**Zyrtec**)

Chlorpheniramine (**Chlor-Trimeton**)

Chlorpromazine (**Thorazine**)

Cimetidine* (**Tagamet**)

Clomipramine (**Anafranil**)

Clorazepate (**Tranxene**)

Clozapine* (**Clozaril**)

Codeine*

Colchicine

Cyclobenzaprine* (**Amrix, Fexmid, Flexeril**)

Cyproheptadine (**Periactin**)

Desipramine* (**Norpramin**)

Dexchlorpheniramine

Dicyclomine (**Bentyl**)

Digoxin (**Lanoxicaps, Lanoxin**)

Diphenhydramine (**Benadryl, Simply Sleep,** etc.)

Fesoterodine (**Toviaz**)

Fluphenazine (**Prolixin**)

Furosemide (**Lasix**)

Hydroxyzine (**Atarax, Vistaril**)

Hyoscyamine (**Anaspaz, Levbid, Levsin, Levsinex, NuLev**)

Imipramine (**Tofranil**)

Loperamide* (**Imodium**)

Loratadine* (**Alavert, Claritin**)

Maprotiline

Meclizine (**Antivert, Bonine**)

Nortriptyline* (**Pamelor**)

Olanzapine* (**Zyprexa**)

Orphenadrine (**Norflex**)

Oxybutynin (**Ditropan**)

Perphenazine (**Trilafon**)

Prochlorperazine* (**Compazine**)

Promethazine (**Phenergan**)

Pseudoephedrine HCl/ Triprolidine HCl*

Thioridazine (**Mellaril**)

Thiothixene (**Navane**)

Tizanidine (**Zanaflex**)

Tolterodine* (**Detrol**)

Trifluoperazine (**Stelazine**)

Trimipramine (**Surmontil**)

* Less severe anticholinergic effects

patients complain about fuzzy thinking, learning problems, or faulty memory while taking drugs like atorvastatin (Lipitor), rosuvastatin (Crestor), or simvastatin (Zocor), such symptoms are frequently dismissed as signs of normal aging. This could be a significant screwup, especially for older people.

Cholesterol is not evil, though drug companies have almost made it seem that way. Without cholesterol, we would die. It is essential for functioning cell membranes. Cholesterol is a building block for hormones like estrogen, testosterone, and vitamin D. The brain contains roughly one-quarter of all the cholesterol in our body. That's because this molecule is indispensable for the formation of the myelin sheath that surrounds nerve cells in the brain and spinal column. Myelin is a little like the insulation that surrounds the wires in your computer or electrical appliances.

We first began to suspect that statins might affect memory and cognition in May 2000, when we received this message from a reader of our newspaper column: "Last fall, my doctor prescribed Lipitor, and after several months I found I was having trouble remembering names and coming up with the right word. At dinner once I said, 'Please pass the elephant,' though I wanted the bread. I told my husband I thought I'd had a stroke. In January a friend came to visit. She was worried about her memory and couldn't think of her daughter's name on the telephone. She, too, was on Lipitor. I asked my doctor to prescribe a different cholesterol medicine. Within a couple of weeks, I was more mentally alert. But my friend (still on Lipitor) was in worse shape and afraid she would lose her job. Her doctor said forgetfulness could not be due to the drug. She finally stopped taking Lipitor anyway and now is much sharper. I am concerned that some people taking Lipitor might think such a reaction was just due to getting older. Is this side effect well known?"

At that time, the answer to the question was a definite no. Most physicians scoffed at the idea that statins could impair cognition. There was nothing in the prescribing information about memory problems or word scrambling. Since then, however, we have received hundreds of comments from people who are convinced that statins caused their confusion and problems with concentration. One woman described this as "big ugly holes burned through my memory."

The most poignant story we have received came from Mike, a retired professor of business law and computer science. He was diagnosed with probable Alzheimer's disease that was progressing very rapidly. He went to his fiftieth college reunion with a sign around his neck that said, "I'm Mike. I have Alzheimer's disease." At his youngest daughter's wedding, he did not recognize people he had known more than twenty years. His decline made it clear that he would soon need long-term nursing care. But then he read about statins and memory problems. After informing his doctor, he discontinued taking simvastatin. Although it took many months, he gradually regained his memory and cognitive ability. When he contacted us, he was back to reading three newspapers a day and was sharp as a tack. A complete neurological workup showed no signs of Alzheimer's disease.

Although there have been no definitive studies of statins and cognition, there are some suggestions that there could be problems. Case reports in the medical literature have begun to crop up.[58-62] And if physicians check the prescribing information, they will find amnesia mentioned with atorvastatin (Lipitor), and memory loss or impairment listed with lovastatin (Mevacor), pravastatin (Pravachol), rosuvastatin (Crestor), and simvastatin (Zocor). We suspect that older people may be especially vulnerable to statin-induced side effects, but until there is better research, all we can recommend is vigilance.

Statins and Mental Function

Beatrice Golomb, MD, PhD, surveyed patients who reported memory or other cognitive problems associated with statins. She published a study titled "Statin-Associated Adverse Cognitive Effects" in 2009. Her findings:

"128 patients (75 percent) experienced cognitive ADRs [adverse drug reactions] determined to be probably or definitely related to statin therapy. Of

143 patients (84 percent) who reported stopping statin therapy, 128 (90 percent) reported improvement in cognitive problems, sometimes within days of statin discontinuation (median time to first-noted recovery 2.5 weeks). Of interest, in some patients, a diagnosis of dementia or Alzheimer's disease reportedly was reversed. Nineteen patients whose symptoms improved or resolved after they discontinued statin therapy and who underwent rechallenge with a statin exhibited cognitive problems again (multiple times in some)!"[63]

Anyone who suspects that a medication is causing memory problems, difficulty with numbers, cognitive impairment, or just plain fuzzy thinking should discuss these concerns with a physician. We certainly don't want anyone to suffer from drug-induced dementia. But we cannot repeat this often enough: no one should *ever* stop medication without consulting a health care professional. Sometimes there is a critical reason for a particular medication, and stopping suddenly could produce disastrous consequences. We hope the top 10 tips below will help guide you or an older friend or relative through that negotiation.

Top 10 Tips to Surviving Old Age

1. Make sure your doctor *likes* older people.
2. Find a good geriatrician.
3. Ask about special dosing requirements.
4. Beware bad drugs (check the Beers List).
5. Avoid anticholinergic drugs if possible.
6. Minimize the number of drugs you take.
7. Seek nondrug treatment when practical.
8. Be assertive.
9. Have an advocate.
10. Stay active.

CHAPTER 11

TOP 10 SCREWUPS PATIENTS MAKE

1. Not telling your story
2. Relying on memory
3. Not doing your homework
4. Skipping instructions
5. Not checking the prescription
6. Trusting all generic drugs
7. Overlooking lifestyle opportunities
8. Not seeking a second opinion
9. Not reading the fine print
10. Not asking for help

Trust but Verify

Most patients trust their physicians, pharmacists, and other health care providers. We certainly do not wish to undermine their faith, but just like any other endeavor, health care is vulnerable to human error. If we assume that our doctors might make snap judgments and miss the correct diagnosis, we may become more assertive in helping them uncover the root cause of our symptoms.

If we recognize that the prescription we get from our physician may not be exactly what the clerk hands us at the drugstore, we may be more conscientious about verifying that the pills, dose, and instructions match what the doctor wrote. If we ask about possible side effects linked to our medications, we may not have to suffer for weeks or months with an avoidable adverse drug reaction. In a word, we all need to take more responsibility for our own health and its care. We can trust our providers to try their best, but we had better be ready to do our homework.

Top 10 Patient Screwups

• **Number one: Not telling your story.** When your doctor knocks, strides into the exam room, and asks you what the problem is, the likelihood is that you will have less than thirty seconds to tell him before you are interrupted.[1-4] Make that time count! Always come to a doctor's appointment prepared. That means bringing a list of things with the most important concerns right at the top. Be assertive and tell your whole story without getting distracted or sidetracked. The only way your doctor can make a proper diagnosis is with all the relevant information.

Take dizziness, for example. Millions suffer with this debilitating symptom. It's hard to diagnose the cause and treat it effectively unless you specialize in neurology or otolaryngology. A primary care provider may be much more interested in discussing cholesterol levels or blood pressure (things he *can* treat) than in addressing the dizziness that is causing you substantial discomfort. Be sure that the doctor understands that if dizziness is your major problem, you don't want to leave until there is some plan of action to deal with it.

Ask the doctor to tell you what she heard you say. Do not leave the doctor's office or let a physician depart your hospital room without confirming that she understood and addressed your primary concerns.

• **Number two: Relying on memory.** Along with your list of most important concerns, make sure to bring a list of *all* prescription and over-the-counter medicines, even if you take them only occasionally, as well as vitamins, minerals, herbs, and dietary supplements. Many people do not think of nutritional supplements as medicines, but each may interact with something else. Trying to remember every single pill you take on the spur of the moment is a challenge not worth taking on. Make a list, including the dose and how often you take your pills, and keep it with you. If that's too complicated, you can always brown-bag it. Just put everything into a bag and take it with you to the appointment. Then make sure your physician actually takes the time to check for interactions or potential side effects that could be causing you trouble. Give her time to look it up on the computer or in a reference book.

Take notes during your appointment. If your doctor has some bad news, the chances are very good that you won't remember very much else. Any instruction or prescription information is likely to be lost in the mental fog that frequently occurs in these situations. If you're not good at taking notes, take along a recording device and ask the doctor if it would be okay for you to record the appointment for future reference so that you won't forget anything important. You could also bring along a family member or friend to take notes for you.

• **Number three: Not doing your homework.** Once upon a time, it was very difficult for any patient to get access to health information. Medical libraries were closed to the general public; you had to have a union card (MD) to get in the door. Many doctors used a Latin code for prescriptions, which created an air of mystery and kept the patient in the dark.

With the Internet, all that is ancient history. If anything, there is an *overabundance* of information. Were you to ask "Dr. Google" about hemorrhoids, you would get nearly 3 million results. Nobody has the time to read through all those links; some, such as MayoClinic.com, provide excellent background information and suggestions about diagnostic possibilities and various treatments, but others do not. Be wary of websites that have lots of pharmaceutical ads. One of the most popular medical websites has been criticized for "pseudomedicine and subtle misinformation . . . that preys on the fear and vulnerability of its users to sell them half-truths and, eventually, pills."[5] There are also lots of websites pushing exotic supplements for hard-to-treat conditions. If the site is primarily trying to sell you something, be skeptical.

It is now possible to search for symptoms, conditions, and a range of therapies from home remedies to prescription drugs. Speaking of medications, you should look up the most common and most serious side effects of the drugs you take. Learn what symptoms to watch out for and when to get in touch with your doctor. Good sources include DailyMed or PubMed (just use Google to find them). These government websites provide valuable resources with no advertising.

Learn all you can about your diagnosis. Make sure your doctor got it right. Ask your doctor how certain she is about this diagnosis, and be sure to ask what else might possibly cause your symptoms. Find out about the short-term prognosis and the possible long-term consequences of the condition. Find out about all of the possible treatment strategies. If various drugs are available, find out which is the most effective and which carries the biggest risk. In our book *Best Choices from the People's Pharmacy,* we did our best to rate treatments for many common conditions based on just such a formula. Your doctor owes it to you to help you evaluate every reasonable option.

Doing your homework also means getting your prescription filled and taking the medicine. If you experience an adverse drug reaction, don't give up on medicine entirely. Another kind of medication might solve the problem without causing complications.

• **Number four: Skipping instructions.** Your doctor really does want to help you get better. A dermatologist who is trying hard to clear up a patient's case of psoriasis becomes understandably frustrated if the drug doesn't work. This becomes even more distressing if the doctor learns the patient is not using the medicine as directed. People with heart failure who don't cut back on salt won't get the results they need. The best doctor-patient relationship is a partnership, and both sides need to pull their weight. We call this participatory medicine, and there is a growing movement to nurture this approach.

• **Number five: Not checking the prescription.** When the doctor hands you a prescription, check it before you leave the office. Make sure it is legible without any Latin codes like *bid* or *hs.* The instructions must be clear and detailed so you can follow them, and they should agree with what your doctor just told you. Don't ask your doctor to fax or phone in a prescription; the opportunity for error is much too high. Ask the nurse or receptionist to make an extra copy of the prescription so you can keep one for your records, or photocopy the prescription before you hand it in to the pharmacy. This way you can check the filled prescription against the printed copy to make sure you received the right drug in the right strength with the precise instructions your doctor gave you. It's a crucial step to catch a drugstore mistake in filling the prescription. Remember, there are at a minimum 50 million dispensing errors each year in this country.[6] When you pick up your pills, don't leave the counter without getting out your copy of the prescription and comparing it to the label on the little bottle. That is how some people have been able to discover that the pharmacist (or possibly the technician) dispensed the wrong drug, or the wrong strength, or gave the wrong instructions.

Pharmacy Faux Pas

"I recently had a prescription filled at my local pharmacy. The dosage was mislabeled big-time. The label read 'take 4 times a day,' but it was supposed to be 4 times a week.

"I caught the error myself before I even left the drugstore. It was lucky that I did.

"I reported the pharmacy mistake to my physician, the state Board of Pharmacy, and the drugstore chain itself."

• **Number six: Trusting all generic drugs.** Once we were among the country's most enthusiastic supporters of generic drugs. We no longer have such blind faith in the ability of the Food and Drug Administration (FDA) to approve or monitor generic drugs.

To use generic drugs sensibly, be sure you know what to expect from your prescription medication. Keep track of objective measures, like blood pressure, blood sugar, or tests for cholesterol, as well as your subjective sense of how you are feeling. As one friend says, "Listen to your body. You're the only one who can." Do not assume that all generics are created equal. Some are fine, but you may not be notified when you are switched from one generic manufacturer to another. You may not realize it until you experience symptoms. If you suspect problems, report them to your doctor and pharmacist and do not accept the assurance that everything is "identical."

• **Number seven: Overlooking lifestyle opportunities.** When you feel sick, you want to get better fast. That makes sense to us and to your doctor. She'll do her best to prescribe medicine that will help you recover. But if you are dealing with a chronic problem, relying on the drugs alone can be a big mistake that leads to more issues later. Just imagine, for example, that you are having difficulties with heartburn (doctors call it dyspepsia). The physician prescribes Nexium or Protonix (proton pump inhibitors [PPIs]), and you go on your merry way, perhaps grumbling a bit about the high price of the pills.

If you stick to this prescription for several months, you may find it quite hard to stop. When you try, your heartburn could well come roaring back. So you stay on the pills for a year or two, or even longer. Many people have. Long-term complications of such medicines include a higher risk of infections (pneumonia as well as a dangerous intestinal infection called *Clostridium difficile*).[7] Other risks include a vulnerability to bone fracture and vitamin B_{12} depletion, which could cause nerve pain and forgetfulness.

For routine heartburn there are far less expensive solutions that are less likely to cause serious side effects. As Dr. Mitchell Katz, director of the San Francisco Department of Public Health, advises, "Once our patients fully appreciate the adverse effects of PPIs, they themselves may prefer other treatments, including tincture of time (many cases of dyspepsia resolve on their own), behavioral changes (e.g., eating smaller meals [especially before bed], weight loss, smoking cessation, stress reduction), and other nonmedical interventions (e.g., raising the head of their bed)."[8]

Heartburn is not the only issue that can be greatly helped with nonmedical approaches. Losing weight can bring blood pressure down surprisingly well, while a combination of dietary changes, red yeast rice, niacin, and psyllium can lower cholesterol. Whenever the doctor suggests a drug that a patient will need indefinitely or "forever," the patient should be asking about other ways to address the problem. Even when the drug is necessary, as insulin is for type 1 diabetes, paying attention to stress management, exercise, and diet can make a huge difference in managing the disease well and reducing the amount of drug therapy needed.

Spice Lowers Blood Pressure

"I accidentally learned that turmeric could help reduce my high blood pressure (160/80) to 140/60. I discovered this by checking my blood pressure after eating an Indian curry.

"My daughter, a nutritionist, advised me to use one-half teaspoon of turmeric daily. I put it in my daily soy shake with a small clove of garlic and fruits. I have now lost weight as well, and my blood pressure usually runs about 120/65."

• **Number eight: Not seeking a second opinion.** If you have ever needed to get your house painted or replace the roof, you have no doubt gone through a process of getting several estimates of what needs to be done and how much it will cost. It's only sensible to make sure that you are not getting fleeced by taking the first offer.

Comparison shopping is much less common in health care. Quite frequently that is because someone else (insurance company, Medicare, health maintenance organization) is paying the bill. On the other hand, you definitely want to make sure you get the right diagnosis and the best recommendation for your treatment. Even if you were paying out of your own pocket, you might not want to have the cheapest surgeon replacing your knee joint. That's why a second opinion is so valuable. Patient safety expert Peter Pronovost, MD, PhD, has told us that more than 100,000 people die as a result of misdiagnosis while in hospitals each year.[9] That does not take into account people who are misdiagnosed in a doctor's office, urgent care clinic, or nursing home. That's why it is so important to ask your primary care physician what else could account for your symptoms. Checking with another physician who will look at your case with fresh eyes is worth the time and effort.

Trust Your Instincts

Jerome Groopman, MD, is the author of many highly regarded books about the practice of medicine. In one of them, *Second Opinions,* he described an experience he and his wife (also an MD) had when his son was a baby. The baby was crying plaintively, wouldn't nurse, had a fever, and was in distress. When he saw black-colored diarrhea, Dr. Groopman knew that "something was wrong."

They took the infant to a local pediatrician, who diagnosed an intestinal virus and sent them on their way with instructions to "keep up the Tylenol."

Their son continued to deteriorate, so eventually these two physician parents took him to the emergency department that evening. The resident who examined him correctly diagnosed a serious intestinal blockage (intussusception) but told the parents that surgery could wait until the morning. Their instincts as parents said otherwise. They sought a second opinion, which led to immediate emergency surgery that saved their baby's life.[10]

We all need to learn an invaluable lesson from Jerome Groopman: trust our intuition and seek a second opinion when the situation calls for it. A defensive doctor may not agree, but assertive action can save lives.

Determining the best treatment for you is not as straightforward as you might imagine. There are dozens of medications for high blood pressure, for example. Finding the one that will be most effective and least likely to cause you unpleasant side effects is often a matter of trial and error. Ask ten different internists for a recommendation, and you might get five or six different opinions. This is even more confusing for a serious condition like cancer. Evaluating the advantages and drawbacks of each treatment is essential for making the right choice.

• **Number nine: Not reading the fine print.** If you have ever made a big purchase such as a car or house, you had to wade through fine print and a legal labyrinth. Trying to make sense of such gobbledygook is daunting. People who were saddled with horrible loans during the housing bust know the devastating consequences of not truly understanding what you are signing.

Anyone who has to go in for a diagnostic or surgical procedure will also be faced with forms to sign. "Informed consent" is a legal requirement before anything important is done to you. You are supposed to understand what is going to happen, along with the benefits and risks. When you sign the form, you give your approval to proceed. The trouble is that most people grant their consent without ever really being fully informed about the medical treatment they are going to receive. When you put lawyer-speak together with doctor-speak, you often end up with information that is incomprehensible.

Uninformed Consent

"Studies show that most patients don't read the forms they sign before undergoing surgery or medical treatment. More than half of those who do read the forms don't understand them, and only a quarter of forms include all of the data patients need to make an informed decision."[11]

Although informed consent is a critical part of doctor-patient communication, most physicians have not been trained on how to make sure the patient truly understands the treatment.[12] Often the doctor rushes through the explanation and may not even have exact statistics on complications at his fingertips. Imagine for a moment that you need a hip or knee replacement. Your orthopedic surgeon can't tell you about the consequences of the specific implant he'll be using because no one actually studies the long-term performance of these devices in a systematic fashion.[13] Most patients would be astonished to learn that the FDA does not require patient testing before it approves artificial joints.

Physicians rarely know the actual effectiveness of the medications they prescribe based on FDA-approved clinical trials. And rarely do they tell patients the actual incidence of common side effects. The only way a doctor can evaluate your knowledge is to have you tell her what you have been told about the medicine or procedure. This "teach-back" technique verifies a true understanding of what has been communicated. Make sure you get answers to all the questions in the sidebar checklist.

Questions to Ask Your Doctor Before Agreeing to Surgery

1. What exactly will be done?
2. Why has it been recommended?
3. What are the alternatives?
4. What kind of anesthesia will be used?
5. What are the pros and cons of the procedure?
6. What are the pros and cons of the anesthesia?
7. What would happen if I opt out of the procedure?
8. What is the name of the doctor or surgeon who will be doing the procedure?
9. Who will be administering the anesthesia?
10. Will there be any other medical staff or learners present?
11. What will they be doing?
12. What are the pros and cons of any medication I will be given?
13. Are there any symptoms that are so serious they require immediate action?

Finally, *never* sign a mediation agreement if you have to go into a hospital for a procedure. Some institutions use these agreements to avoid litigation. Many patients don't realize they are signing away their right to sue if something horrible happens. They also may fear that if they don't sign a mediation agreement, the procedure won't be done. That is usually not true.

• **Number ten: Not asking for help.** Never go to the hospital alone. There are so many opportunities for misadventure that you should always have an advocate with you 24/7. That means family and friends will need to create a schedule so that you will have someone with you at all times. If you cannot arrange to have a volunteer, you may want to pay for a private-duty nurse who can serve that function. Whoever is there with you needs to double-check everything that happens. That means all tests, medications, procedures, and anything else that is done to you. That person will need to squawk like hell if something doesn't seem right. Remember, at least one mistake will probably be made every day you are hospitalized.[14]

A brilliant physician we know who serves at the highest level of a top-notch hospital confided to us that this concept is crucial. He himself served as the patient advocate for his father. During the hospital stay, a number of errors were averted because the physician son was vigilant.

Even if you are not in the hospital, having an extra pair of eyes and ears with you at a doctor visit can be extremely useful. You may forget to ask a crucial question that a partner can remember. Or you may not hear what the doctor is telling you, especially if it is bad news. A diagnosis of heart disease, cancer, or Alzheimer's disease can be so traumatic that everything else the doctor says from that moment on will be a blur. Someone who can take notes or record the conversation can help you figure out how to proceed after the visit is over.

CHAPTER 12

CLOSING THE COMMUNICATION CHASM

Doubtless you have heard the phrase "Men are from Mars; women are from Venus." The chasm between patients and health care providers is often even wider. Patients come to the encounter feeling vulnerable, powerless, and dependent on the doctor. They tell the physician some of their most personal secrets and reveal things they would never tell a friend or even a family member. They may come to think of their physician almost as a confidant or a friend. If the health issue is a serious one, they may be hoping that the doctor can act as a champion or savior. From the patient's perspective, the relationship feels intensely intimate and extremely important. In most cases, the patient has only one or, at most, a few doctors.

The physician, on the other hand, has many patients (often thousands seen over the course of a year or two) and has probably heard similar stories, personal though they may be. Although the doctor may care deeply about her patients, the relationship does not feel so intimate from her perspective. She will do her best to help the patient get well, but it is part of her job. The patient encounter is just one of many she will have during the day, while for the patient this doctor visit is usually the only one of the day, and perhaps of the month or year.

Wait Time

Unless doctors and patients can put themselves in the other's shoes—a difficult trick—there are going to be points of friction. Just think about one common problem: wait time. Patients complain about time spent waiting more often than almost any other aspect of health care. An article in the *Wall Street Journal* by Melinda Beck describes the average wait time in 2010 as about twenty-two minutes.[1] No surprise: the longer patients wait, the less satisfied they are with the entire visit. Nor should it surprise anyone that doctors also hate to wait. But here *is* a surprise: they, too, must wait for patients more often than they would like.

One busy hospital-based practice conducted a patient flow study to help them make their practice more efficient. Reducing patient wait times was also a goal, but first they needed to find out how long patients waited and at what points in the process. The patient flow study showed that patients generally arrived about twenty minutes before appointment time. This was a surprise to the doctors, who had the impression patients were often late. It turns out, though, that the process of checking in, having vital signs measured, reviewing medications, and being led to an exam room often took more than thirty minutes. You don't have to be a mathematical genius to figure out that means the doctors were indeed waiting for the first patient of the day. And with patients scheduled back-to-back, even a brief initial delay tends to multiply over the course of the day, until doctors are far behind and struggling by late afternoon, with patients waiting far longer than twenty minutes. Both sides felt that the other side was to blame, while, in truth, those waits were really due mostly to the way the system was set up.

What can patients do about this? It may help, as Melinda Beck suggests in the *Wall Street Journal*, to request the first appointment of the day or the first one after lunch. Health care providers are less likely to have fallen behind at those times. Ask how far ahead you should arrive for your appointment; then be on time. It turns out that both patients who arrive extremely early and those who arrive extremely late can throw the doctor's schedule out of kilter.* If you make either behavior

---

* Probably everyone understands why latecomers mess up the schedule. But it is not intuitive why the early birds could, too. Here's the story: Imagine you arrive at 10:00 for your 11:00 A.M. appointment because you like to be early. The staff sees you sitting there, and somewhere around 10:15 or 10:20 they put you in an exam room because they hate it when patients have to be in the waiting room so long. At 10:25, the patient with the 10:30 appointment arrives. But there is no room for him, because you are there. As a result, you'll be seen first, and that patient will wait a long time, despite being on time for his appointment.

a regular habit, the office staff may find ways to discourage your be-havior, and you may feel, quite reasonably, that you are being punished.

Waiting for Dr. Godot

"My brother waited and waited for his doctor—first in the waiting room, then in the exam room. Eventually, when *no one* came in to check on him, he went to the front desk. *The doctor had left and gone home!*

"Laughable. My brother really likes the doctor. I spoke to the same doctor while taking a friend to see him and told him how much my brother thought of him and brought up my brother's being left behind. The doctor told me that it happens and then went on to tell me about a patient who had been delivered to his office from a nursing home. He was placed in an exam room to wait. The cleaning crew found the man that night after everyone had left the office. I swear, I did not make this up!"

It's not against the rules to politely inquire, if you have been sitting in the exam room for thirty or forty minutes, when you might expect the doctor to be in. That might save you from being forgotten. Of course, if you've had to dress in a paper exam robe that opens in the back, you may not want to wander around the office very far. If that's the case, you might suggest that the practice adopt exam gowns that tie in front, like a bathrobe.

Communication Style

Patients tend to resent a condescending tone of voice from the doctor. A dear friend who is sharp and savvy said that she is tired of being talked to as if she were twelve. Patients don't have the same knowledge as doc-tors, to be sure, but most are capable of understanding their situation if it is put in ordinary language. Some doctors like to throw around big words and abbreviations, perhaps as a matter of habit. Asking for clarification is a good way to counter the vocabulary problem, though it may do nothing for the tone of voice. Doctors may worry if a patient doesn't ask any question because they can't tell if the patient has understood. It's a good idea to try to summarize what the doctor has said, especially with respect to the treatment ("I should take one of these pills three times a day, at mealtime, is that right?") just to confirm you've got it.

Come prepared for your visit. If there is a specific issue troubling you, bring the notes on the exact symptoms, when they occur, how long they last, and any other details that seem relevant so you can be as clear as possible. If it is a more general visit, bring a list of your top three questions so you and the provider can go over them together. Try to make sure that the most serious issue is right at the top of the list. (Doctors really hate being surprised with "one more thing, Doctor," as they are going out the door.) If you are good at taking notes, bring a notepad. If not, bring a relative, friend, or recording device. Ask your doctor first if she minds you using the tape recorder, cell phone, or other device to make sure that you have her complete answers and instructions and can consult them later. A reasonable doctor should be pleased.

Power Struggle

Doctors spend years in medical school, residency, and specialist training, so they tend to get annoyed with patients who seem to think they know what is wrong with them and how it should be treated. The emotional reaction to this situation tends to be framed as: "I'm the doctor here. Who do you think you are?"

While patients don't have the same knowledge base as doctors, they do have their own areas of expertise: they have lived in their own bodies all their lives, and they know how those bodies feel and, often, how they react to certain medications or situations. This is especially true of patients with chronic diseases. As one of our friends with cystic fibrosis says, "The doctor is the expert on the disease, but I am the expert on my body." When a patient and a doctor can acknowledge each other's areas of expertise and work together, the outcome is likely to be much more satisfactory than when feathers get ruffled.

When Mother Knows Best

"I hate condescending doctors. There was a time when my son, who has hydrocephalus, was having symptoms of a blocked shunt. I took him to a neurosurgeon at the hospital (his neurosurgeon wasn't in, but this doctor was the head of the practice). They took all the necessary CTs [computerized tomography scans], X-rays, et cetera, and according to this neurosurgeon, all looked okay. So he patted me on the shoulder and said, 'Everything is fine, but we'll keep him in overnight for you, Mom.'

"Well, at three in the morning, his heart rate dropped, and he went into a hydrocephalus coma. They had to do emergency surgery!"

Researchers have found that communication problems are responsible for a fair amount of unnecessary suffering. Experts who have studied patient reactions to prescription drugs concluded that the severity or the duration of many of these reactions could be reduced significantly if doctors told patients what to watch for and asked patients about their medication-related symptoms.[2] Patients need to remember that doctors can't read minds. To be able to address a drug side effect, the doctor must be told about it. Here again, specificity is a great help.

Communication problems between professionals can also cause difficulty. Sometimes the doctor writing a prescription for a medication or an imaging study will slip up. With luck, the pharmacist or the radiologist will catch an odd-looking prescription and question it. The degree to which this assistance is welcomed varies considerably from doctor to doctor. Questioning or confirming the doctor's orders becomes more complicated when clerical personnel have to act as the middlemen. There may be little or nothing a patient can do about this type of communication gap, but it always makes sense to ask the doctor to explain exactly what she intends and why. That may allow for appropriate interpretation or intervention if there is a question about the prescription itself.

Keeping Records

Doctors are not auto mechanics. They need patients' involvement to help them do their best work. If you have a chronic health condition, you need to keep track of vital statistics. This may mean monitoring blood pressure every week or measuring blood sugar several times a day. The patient and the doctor together should agree on what metrics are helpful and how often they should be done. If you don't understand why a certain measurement would be needed so often, request an explanation. It might not occur to you that just weighing yourself every morning could give the doctor an excellent clue on how you are doing with your heart failure regimen. It might not seem important, but it could be vital.

If you are seeing the doctor for a new problem, make sure you have a succinct summary of your symptoms, including when they occur and how long they last. This can be crucial for the doctor trying to figure out a diagnosis. The doctor definitely needs to know all the medicines you take (including over-the-counter products and supplements), either in a written list or bundled up in a brown bag.

Web Wrangling

Misunderstandings are especially common when it comes to Internet research. From the doctor's perspective, the patient who arrives armed with reams of printouts and a specific diagnosis or treatment plan in mind doesn't seem to value the doctor's skills.

From the patient's perspective, the doctor who dismisses her concerns is putting her down. If the patient has used good sense and brought in only information that is relevant to her case, discussing the alternatives she has uncovered won't waste anyone's time and may even offer some ideas the doctor hasn't considered. At the very least, the patient should go away with a better understanding of her condition and a sense of partnership, which will not happen if the doctor acts resentful. Mutual respect is essential to this partnership.

Follow-up

Follow-up is a two-way street. The doctor expects that the patient will fill the prescription or follow the recommendation that has been given and will report back on progress—or particularly on lack of progress! Patients who don't take their medicine or show up for physical therapy do not give themselves the best chance for recovery. If you have tried your doctor's suggestion and you're not getting better or your symptoms are even worsening, don't wait for the next scheduled visit. Get in touch with the doctor and make your report. She may want you to come in sooner.

The doctor, on the other hand, also has follow-up obligations. One is to respond to your question or report. To make this easier, ask the doctor how he prefers to get such messages. Some doctors are comfortable using e-mail. Those who have tried it often find it helps cut down on phone tag and is helpful and efficient rather than burdensome.[3-6] It makes sense to get the expectations clear on both sides: patients should not e-mail doctors about emergencies (call 911). Doctors should let patients know how long it is likely to take for a response. And everyone should keep in mind that e-mail is not infallible: sometimes a message you send doesn't get through.

Other doctors or patients prefer a phone call. Here, too, however, clear expectations on both sides are helpful. If the issue is urgent, make sure the person answering the phone understands that. Otherwise, be prepared to wait until the doctor has an opportunity to get back in touch with you.

The doctor's other responsibility on follow-up is to give you the results of tests and explain the implications to you. When the doctor orders a test, ask when you should expect to learn about the results. Put it on your calendar, and if you don't hear by the expected date, make a call. Then add the results to your personal record so you can keep track of what is going on with your health.

Keeping Track

"I started accumulating my personal medical information in earnest about ten years ago and aggressively maintaining it about five years ago. It's not easy, but it can be done. Lab results are especially tricky but important.

"The net of all this effort is that I now have a rather complete record, with several variables (e.g., blood pressure, cholesterol, PSA [prostate-specific antigen]) graphed over time for quick analysis. When my PSA started to rise quickly, it was easy to see and resulted in early confirmation and cure of prostate cancer. I take the complete history with me to every medical appointment, with a summary that I can give the provider.

"This shows that one can take the trouble to develop and maintain a complete history on one's own. It may actually help in some instances. It's a fun exercise, and you will die leaving a well-documented, if not beautiful, body."

Coordinating Care

A patient who sees more than one doctor may assume that they all communicate with one another. That is often not the case. Even when the primary doctor refers the patient to a specialist, the report that comes back may be incomplete, or it may go astray. To the extent possible, patients may need to be their own "air traffic controllers," keeping track of all the tests, reports, recommendations, and prescriptions. They may need to summarize this record for the primary care provider so nothing gets overlooked. If the patient gets left out of the loop, a physician who doesn't touch base with any of the other health care providers involved can make that patient feel extremely frustrated! Don't let it happen to you.

Assessing Alternatives

Assessing alternatives is an area fraught with potential conflict between doctors and patients. Doctors vary in their knowledge of and openness to herbal medicine, dietary supplements, and other alternative approaches. If the patient senses that the doctor will respond with scorn, he's likely to keep his dietary supplement regimen a secret. In the past, doctors would sneer about "expensive urine" if a patient was taking vitamins. The evidence on alternative approaches (just like the evidence on certain medications) doesn't always hold up well. But if something might help and won't hurt, it may be worth a try. If the patient wants to try meditation to help ease presurgical anxiety, why not? Even if the doctor doesn't know the research, discouraging such an apparently benign practice seems unproductive.

On the other hand, a patient who is adamant about an untested and highly unusual treatment instead of the Food and Drug Administration–approved medicine that the doctor prescribed can expect a weary sigh, at best. To keep from aggravating the provider, a patient interested in an alternative approach should do the homework. Look up the research (that means, of course, go beyond the websites selling the product), bring in the best summary, and negotiate with the doctor. A patient might, for example, request three months for a trial of diet, exercise, and red yeast rice to lower cholesterol before starting on a statin. Having a copy of the clinical trial[7] reported in a medical journal showing that this approach can work is a plus.

Top 10 Tips to Promote Good Communication

1. Find out when to arrive.
2. Be on time.
3. Ask for clarification of diagnoses and treatments.
4. Take notes.
5. Be clear about your previous treatment experience (know your body).
6. Keep records.
7. Target Web research carefully.
8. Follow up on test results.
9. Coordinate your other doctors' recommendations.
10. Do the homework on alternative approaches.

CHAPTER 13

TOP SCREWUPS IN COMMON CONDITIONS

There is a dynamic tension in medicine that is rarely discussed in public. For the most part, health care providers try to present themselves as one big happy family getting along harmoniously and working together seamlessly. Not surprisingly, the truth can be quite different.

The Forest and the Trees

Specialists make more than generalists. Researchers have estimated that cardiologists, for example, earn on average over $400,000 annually. Primary care physicians, on the other hand, make about half that much.[1] Not surprisingly, that kind of income disparity influences medical students in the choices they make. Specialists are also treated with greater respect in many situations, especially by hospital administrators and office managers. Understandably, this sometimes generates resentment from the generalist, who may feel that he or she can handle certain conditions well and doesn't see a value in specialist care for straightforward conditions.

Once upon a time, primary care providers (PCPs) were called GPs, or general practitioners. They delivered babies, performed minor surgeries, and treated a wide range of common conditions. They even made house calls. Today our frontline providers are nurse practitioners (NPs), physician assistants (PAs), family practice doctors, internists, and pediatricians. Like the old GP, they are good at seeing the big picture. They get to know the patient and often the family. They are supposed to have the time to better understand how a certain condition is affecting the whole body, not just a single organ. In other words, how does a patient's asthma affect his ability to exercise and work? What impact does it have on emotional well-being and family life? A specialist may be more concerned about lung function than drug side effects, but aggressive treatment can have unforeseen and devastating complications.

Primary care providers can encourage people to quit smoking and lose weight and may be able to coach them to success. Specialists may not have time for such seemingly mundane efforts. Since PCPs have the bird's-eye view, they can help the patient evaluate a range of options for treating conditions like diabetes, high blood pressure, or insomnia. There is no single one-size-fits-all treatment that is exactly right for everyone, so the generalist can help each patient sort through several approaches. Someone with many different conditions could easily see more than one specialist, such as a gastroenterologist, a cardiologist, a dermatologist, and a rheumatologist. Each is concerned primarily with the issues regarding his or her expertise. The primary care provider can help make sure that the various recommendations and prescribed medications don't conflict with one another.

Seeing the big picture is extremely valuable, but occasionally important details may get missed. For example, a nurse practitioner or a family practice physician may assume that moderate leg pain after an exercise workout is caused by a muscle strain rather than a life-threatening blood clot (deep vein thrombosis [DVT]). Abdominal discomfort, bloating, constipation, and/or diarrhea may be attributed to IBS (irritable bowel syndrome), whereas it could actually be ovarian cancer. Knowing how to distinguish between a recurrent cough brought on by allergies or postnasal drip rather than a medication or lung cancer is essential.

Tunnel Vision

Instead of gazing at the forest, the specialist is an expert on a particular tree. She may be a pediatric neurologist specializing in children's epilepsy. Not only will this kind of physician be better able to diagnose the precise kind of seizure disorder a child may be suffering, she will also be better prepared to determine the best treatment with the fewest side effects. There are many times when that sort of in-depth expertise is essential.

An otolaryngologist (ear, nose, and throat specialist) may be able to diagnose dizziness caused by benign paroxysmal positional vertigo (BPPV). Older people frequently develop symptoms of dizziness when they change their head position. If they look up or roll over in bed, an attack can be triggered. The symptoms of BPPV are caused by calcium carbonate crystals that have migrated within an ear canal. These crystals can often be repositioned with a simple series of head movements (the Epley maneuver). A neurologist or audiologist trained in Epley can perform this little trick in about ten minutes and help someone who has been miserable for months walk out of the office cured. A primary care provider who is uncertain about BPPV might send the patient home with an ineffective prescription to treat vertigo.

Specialists are seductive. They have spent extra years studying a particular area and are often portrayed as the final authority for a specific ailment. It is hardly surprising that patients seek out such expertise, especially if they have had an unsatisfactory experience with their primary care provider. But there are limitations to specialist care. An endocrinologist may be very knowledgeable about a particular problem, such as diabetes, and a cardiologist may understand the intricacies of cholesterol. Nevertheless, focusing on such a narrow problem can create other complications down the road. A diabetes expert who treats patients aggressively to get blood sugar into the normal range may actually endanger their health. Such "tight" control can lead to hypoglycemia (low blood sugar), which can be life threatening.[2]

A cardiologist who sees high cholesterol as the enemy and cholesterol-lowering statins as the solution may be so enthralled with improved lipid levels that he dismisses statin-induced muscle pain that interferes with a person's ability to exercise. A primary care provider may realize that exercising and socializing are as important as lowering cholesterol. Trading short-term gain in the form of great lab numbers for long-term pain is not necessarily a good outcome. A specialist may solve one problem only to create others that different doctors will have to deal with decades later. For example, statins such as atorvastatin (Lipitor) or simvastatin (Zocor) may increase the risk of cataracts down the road.[3]

The Team Solution

The patient must take responsibility for balancing the expertise of the specialist with the oversight of the primary care provider. We need both primary care providers and specialists working together cooperatively and communicating clearly to serve the patient's best interests. Each needs to know his or her own limits and to be able to set aside ego in order to avoid missteps. The patient needs to know when to ask for a second opinion or greater expertise. We suggest starting with the primary care provider and moving on to a specialist only if the condition does not seem to be improving with treatment. When a primary care provider senses that the initial diagnosis may not be correct or that the patient is not responding as expected, a referral is a good idea.

Avoiding Common Screwups for Common Conditions

The goal of this section is to alert you to a few of the errors you should watch for when you are being treated for a common condition. Medical students spend a lot of their extensive education learning what to do about extremely rare and unusual conditions. But what bothers most people most of the time are common problems. Many of these are considered easy to treat, but there are some mistakes that providers make frequently.

Some of our recommendations for how to sidestep errors are common sense, while others have been distilled from the literature and our interviews with top experts on our radio show, *The People's Pharmacy*. We hope you'll find a lot of helpful suggestions on how to protect yourself when you are dealing with common ailments. Ultimately, though, your physician knows your situation far better than anyone else. This book cannot substitute for the medical advice or care of a physician. The reader must consult a doctor in matters relating to his or her health, especially with regard to any signs or symptoms that may require diagnosis or medical attention. Any health problems that do not get better promptly or that get worse should be evaluated and treated by an appropriate clinician.

ACNE

Acne is so well known that it hardly needs to be described. Outbreaks of pimples are especially common among adolescents and sometimes even younger children, but acne is not at all unusual among adults. Surprisingly, though, the exact cause of acne is incompletely understood. Oil-producing hair follicles may become blocked with dead skin cells or excess oil. Certain bacteria *(Propionibacterium acnes)* that live on the skin may contribute to the inflammation of these pores, which seems to lead to zits. Hormonal imbalance and excess oil production also appear to contribute to the condition. Occasionally, acne can be traced to drug reactions. It is important to get the doctor's best estimate of what factors are contributing to the breakouts so that treatment can be focused where it is most likely to help.[1]

It is important for an adult with pimples and redness to ask the doctor whether the skin condition is acne or rosacea, sometimes called acne rosacea just for confusion. Although the bumps may look similar, the treatment is different.

The first line of treatment for mild acne with whiteheads and blackheads and very few angry red inflamed pustules is a topical retinoid (vitamin A derivatives) such as tretinoin (Altinac, Atralin, Avita, Retin-A); adapalene (Differin); or tazarotene (Tazorac).[2] If a mild case of acne has predominantly red inflamed bumps, the doctor might suggest benzoyl peroxide in addition. Benzoyl peroxide is available over the counter as well as by prescription under a large number of brand names.[3] For moderate acne, a topical antibiotic might be added to the benzoyl peroxide. In severe cystic acne, the drug of choice may be isotretinoin. Because this medication can cause birth defects, any woman who takes it undergoes pregnancy testing first and is exhorted to use effective contraception. Sometimes, in fact, oral contraceptives themselves may be used to treat moderate acne,[4] either alone or in combination with the topical therapies mentioned.[5]

A study in Australia found that primary care providers don't always follow the guidelines for managing acne,[6] but many of them do quite a good job. One of the mistakes that they may make is to rely on antibiotics, either topical or oral, for too long a period of time. The bacteria associated with acne can develop resistance,[7] and then the antibiotic is no longer effective. Pairing a topical antibiotic with benzoyl peroxide may discourage resistance, but the best protection is to avoid overuse.[8] Clindamycin, an antibiotic that dermatologists once prescribed routinely, might be the most dramatic example of the hazards of overuse.[9] Resistance to clindamycin has appeared in *Clostridium difficile,* a microbe that causes a very nasty and sometimes life-threatening diarrhea. Overuse of the antibiotic may have contributed to the current resurgence of this dangerous infection.

Another very common screwup is the denial that diet can affect the skin. Back in 1969, dermatologists wrote that the claims that eating too much carbohydrate or fat would affect the skin were unproven[10] (and, by implication, urban legends). Dermatologists defended this view vociferously at least until the turn of the twenty-first century,[11] viewing patients' beliefs that diet might be involved as misconceptions that needed to be debunked.[12]

Over the past several years, however, the evidence has been accumulating that a diet high in glycemic load (lots of refined and processed carbohydrates like bagels, bread, cake, cookies, or crackers) could contribute to blemishes.[13-14] The problem seems to be the insulin response to these carbohydrates and even milk products.[15-16] One researcher has hypothesized that isotretinoin works by reversing the effects of insulin-triggered growth factor activation at the level of cellular nuclei.[17] Switching to a low-glycemic-load diet with lots of vegetables and fruits and very few refined carbohydrates may require attention, but it is neither expensive nor dangerous, and it might have other health benefits over the long term. To learn more about how to do this, you'll find details in books such as *The New Glucose Revolution* or *The Low GI Handbook*, both by Jennie Brand-Miller, MD, and her colleagues.

To protect yourself from errors in the treatment of acne, it is critical to take the time to understand the benefits and the risks of the prescription your doctor is offering. This conversation might even take more than one session, particularly if the treatment, like oral isotretinoin, has considerable risks. It could be a mistake to fail to consider a treatment that might clear up cystic acne for years, but it is foolish not to educate yourself on the potential problems. Do ask the doctor about the likelihood of those problems, and be alert for them if you decide to use the drug. But even before you make that decision, also ask the physician about the likelihood that you will experience benefit from the treatment.

ALZHEIMER'S DISEASE

Alzheimer's disease is one of the most dreaded diagnoses a person can receive. It conjures up the image of an older person who can't find her way home from the market or even remember whether she ate lunch and who doesn't recognize beloved family members. The first person to be diagnosed with Alzheimer's disease was a woman whose memory and speech began to fail in her early fifties. She had become disoriented, confused, and paranoid and couldn't manage simple household tasks such as cooking when her husband had her committed to a mental institution in November 1901.[1] A physician at the institution, Dr. Alois Alzheimer, became interested in her case. When she died, in 1906, he examined her brain under the microscope and discovered the plaques and the neurofibrillary tangles that are the identifying characteristics of the disease that was named in his honor.

A definitive diagnosis of Alzheimer's disease can be made only after the patient dies, through an examination of the brain. There are tests that can determine a high probability of Alzheimer's disease; nonetheless, a number of conditions mimic this dementia but could be reversed with proper treatment. The top screwup in treating Alzheimer's disease is to fail to rule out other causes of memory problems and peculiar behavior. These may be present in 10 to 25 percent of the patients who develop symptoms of dementia, such as trouble thinking and managing activities of daily life.[2]

Dementia from Antidepressants

"I found that dosages or drugs that may be fine if you are fifty or sixty may be very dangerous as you get older unless the dosages or the drugs are changed. I was seventy when I was diagnosed with dementia by a neurologist (moderate dementia with Alzheimer's symptoms). This was after a year of losing my memory and my sense of balance. I was so far gone that the diagnosis meant little to me, although it was crushing to my family.

"I was taking several prescribed antidepressants (Zoloft and Wellbutrin) plus Neurontin [for pain]. My daughter, a nurse who had studied Neurontin, was convinced the problem was due to an interaction of Neurontin with the antidepressants.

"My doctor, a psychiatrist, reduced the Neurontin, and I was better within a few days. By the time the Neurontin was phased out completely, I was back to normal. I suspect that many older people, especially in nursing homes, have similar problems that aren't discovered."

By the time a person is undergoing evaluation for possible Alzheimer's disease, he or she may not be capable of managing the interaction with the physician. Sometimes, though, patients get very good at "covering" their deficits in a casual social situation. That means you, the family member, or close friend, will need to insist that the doctor make sure the problems are not due to an underactive thyroid gland, serious depression, B vitamin deficiency, celiac disease, diabetes, dehydration, infection, liver failure, or even adverse drug reactions. Any of these could cause symptoms similar to those of Alzheimer's disease, and many of them could be ameliorated with appropriate treatment. It is also important to pay attention to health crises before a person has obvious signs of Alzheimer's disease: older people hospitalized with a serious blood infection (sepsis) are significantly more likely to develop cognitive impairment if they survive.[3]

Celiac Disease and Dementia

"I had heard of celiac disease, but I did not know it could show up in adulthood. I figured I had nothing to lose by eliminating wheat from my diet for a while.

"After a week of rice and vegetables, I couldn't believe how much better I felt. The bloating, gas, diarrhea, and puffiness were gone. Best of all, though, the depression, lethargy, and inability to concentrate and think began to lift.

"Not long before, I had insisted my doctor test me for Alzheimer's! I was losing my ability to recognize faces. I couldn't have written this letter because I wouldn't have been able to sustain a train of thought long enough to get past the first paragraph."

A diagnosis of Alzheimer's disease should not be made on the basis of a single short visit or by means of a simple checklist. A careful history is a crucial starting point for making a diagnosis. Talking with family members about behavioral patterns and how they change over time is almost always helpful. If possible, this "family member history" should be done independently of the patient. According to psychiatrist Murali Doraswaimy, MD, and social worker Lisa Gwyther, MSW, the following symptoms raise red flags and should trigger further investigation, since the underlying cause might not be Alzheimer's:[4]

- Tingling and numbness of hands or feet
- Muscle twitches or profound weakness
- Slurred speech
- Bladder control problems
- Gasping for breath while asleep
- Poor balance

- Extreme sensitivity to cold
- Deep apathy or preoccupation with death
- Sudden onset of memory loss with very rapid decline
- Recent heart or lung surgery
- Irregular heart rhythm
- Recent stroke, uncontrolled high blood pressure, diabetes, excess

drinking, recent infection

Another screwup that is made with people who seem to have Alzheimer's disease is to wait until some health crisis triggers institutionalization and then treat the patients as nursing home management problems with high-powered antipsychotic drugs such as haloperidol (Haldol) or olanzapine (Zyprexa). Although these drugs are used to calm agitated patients, they are not approved for this purpose, and the Food and Drug Administration warns that these medications increase the risk of imminent death in elderly patients with dementia.[5] Unfortunately, other methods of defusing agitation or behavioral problems in patients with dementia are labor-intensive, time consuming, and not always effective.[6] No drugs have been approved for treating distressed or unruly patients with Alzheimer's disease or other dementia.

There are prescription medicines for treating Alzheimer's disease. These include such medications as donepezil (Aricept), galantamine (Razadyne), and rivastigmine (Exelon). These drugs are supposed to work by slowing the breakdown of acetylcholine, a brain chemical that neurons use to communicate among themselves. The theory is elegant, but the practical results are less than dazzling. A fourth drug, memantine (Namenda), acts on a different brain chemical. Because of that, it is sometimes prescribed in combination with one of the others.[7] There do not seem to be significant differences in efficacy among the various drugs used to treat this disease.[8]

Although we cannot characterize a prescription for one of these drugs as an error, it isn't as helpful as one might wish. An important long-term, double-blind study of donepezil (Aricept) found that people taking the drug did not have a significant delay in the need for nursing home care compared to those on placebo.[9] The researchers concluded: "Donepezil is not cost effective, with benefits below minimally relevant thresholds. More effective treatments than Cholinesterase inhibitors are needed for Alzheimer's disease."[10] Two separate Cochrane reviews that evaluated placebo-controlled and head-to-head studies of these drugs found that they modestly slowed cognitive decline and were somewhat helpful for activities of daily living.[11-12] The drugs can cause side effects, particularly nausea, vomiting, diarrhea, and loss of appetite. When the doctor prescribes any of these drugs, expect to take several weeks, at a minimum, to build up to the appropriate dose.

Watch out for another common screwup: a prescription for a medicine to control overactive bladder, such as tolterodine (Detrol), oxybutynin (Ditropan) or fesoterodine (Toviaz), may counteract any potential benefit from the cholinesterase inhibitor.[13] These and many other drugs, such as diphenhydramine (Benadryl, Tylenol PM) or meclizine (Antivert, Bonine) for dizziness are anticholinergic drugs—using exactly the opposite biochemical action as the Alzheimer's disease drugs (see the list of such drugs on page 164). Just as it doesn't make sense to drive with a foot on the brake and one on the gas, it doesn't make sense to mix antagonistic medications. Ask the doctor if the drug being prescribed is "anticholinergic." If so, ask which is more important: the new anticholinergic medicine or the Alzheimer's treatment. Do not use them together for any significant period of time without a compelling reason.

ARTHRITIS

Osteoarthritis has most likely afflicted human beings for millennia. Paleoanthropologists commonly find evidence of arthritis in the skeletal remains of people from the Neolithic era.[1] Despite the accumulated years of experience with the condition, however, nobody seems to have come up with a brilliant solution.

There certainly are plenty of people who would welcome one. According to the Arthritis Foundation, an estimated 27 million Americans suffer from joint pain and stiffness due to osteoarthritis.[2] Although there are many different types of arthritis, and different treatments that appear to be most appropriate for them, osteoarthritis is the most common, and the one that probably accounts for the majority of sore joints.

The biggest mistake that a person with arthritis could make is to stop moving. It's certainly a temptation when the joints hurt to avoid painful activity. But finding some moderate-level exercise that is tolerable and practicing it regularly is one of the best ways to maintain the ability to use the joint. It's no wonder, though, that people have been eager to try new treatments that offer the promise of pain relief and better function.

Back in the 1950s, doctors were enthusiastic about cortisone and other drugs in the same category. These anti-inflammatory steroids were especially effective in relieving the pain of rheumatoid arthritis, an autoimmune condition in which the body attacks its own joint tissue. At first, patients loved the relief they got from drugs like dexamethasone or prednisone. But the long-term side effects of these corticosteroids are devastating. They can lead to bone loss, weight gain, cataracts, glaucoma, high blood pressure, fluid retention, thinner skin, stomach ulcers, impaired wound healing, greater susceptibility to infection, and a host of other problems. As a result of this side effect profile, corticosteroids are reserved for special situations rather than as a regular treatment for arthritic joints.

Instead, doctors turned to *nonsteroidal* anti-inflammatory drugs (NSAIDs). Despite the fancy name and the fact that they started out as powerful prescription medicines, NSAIDs are among the most familiar and popular products in the pharmacy. Ibuprofen (Advil, Motrin, etc.) is a sterling example. So is naproxen (Aleve). Both are sold in huge quantities without a prescription. So is aspirin. This was actually the first NSAID on the market, back in 1899, even before the term *NSAID* was invented. Overlooking aspirin and using an expensive prescription NSAID like celecoxib (Celebrex) or meloxicam (Mobic) is a mistake for anyone who can tolerate aspirin. Aspirin, despite its lowly image, is unsurpassed as an anti-inflammatory pain reliever and has side benefits in helping to protect against blood clots that cause deadly heart attacks and strokes.[3-5] Aspirin use also appears to lower the risk of a number of common cancers.[6-8]

Aspirin does have dangers, however, and the doctor should be monitoring for possible digestive tract irritation, ulcers, and bleeding in a patient using aspirin for pain relief. Some people are allergic to aspirin and must avoid it completely. Others take medicines that interact badly with this pain reliever. Taking aspirin without paying attention to the potential hazards could be a serious screwup. The same range of adverse effects holds true for the NSAIDs as well, whether they are over the counter, like ibuprofen and naproxen, or prescription only, such as diclofenac (Cataflam, Voltaren) or etodolac (Lodine). An estimated 100,000 hospitalizations and 16,000 deaths a year have been attributed to gastrointestinal bleeding from ulcers caused by aspirin or NSAIDs.[9]

All this tends to leave people with arthritis feeling rather desperate. It is little wonder that when rofecoxib (Vioxx) and comparable drugs were developed, patients and doctors alike were enthusiastic. Although there never was any evidence that Vioxx offered more effective pain relief, people were hopeful. Doctors were convinced that the digestive tract protection such drugs were supposed to provide would be well worthwhile. It wasn't until years later that studies revealed these drugs increased the risk of dying from heart attacks and strokes.[10-11]

What can someone do for joint pain that undermines the quality of life? Despite the problems with NSAID pills, it is possible to use NSAIDs topically. They may kick in a bit more slowly with pain relief, but after two or three weeks, the relief they offer is pretty similar.[12] The Food and Drug Administration has approved three forms of diclofenac to be applied to the skin on or near the sore joint: Voltaren Gel, Flector patch, and Pennsaid Topical Solution. Putting medicine on the skin might trigger a rash in sensitive individuals, but it is less likely to cause serious digestive tract problems.[13] Adverse reactions are still possible, so patients using one of these topical pain medicines need to stay in touch with their physicians.[14]

Another approach that the doctor may offer a desperate patient is a steroid injection into the joint. Although this treatment often eases pain in the short term, it does not provide reliable long-term relief for tendinitis.[15] Steroid injections may offer many patients relief from arthritis joint pain for a few months, but the pain relief appears to fade more quickly with each subsequent injection.[16] If a steroid injection seems to be the best option to calm a painful joint, request that it be done under ultrasound guidance.[17] This helps ensure that the medication gets where it belongs. Keep in mind, though, that corticosteroids can weaken tendons. So while an injection may occasionally be a helpful tactic, getting repeated shots into a sore joint for diminishing pain relief might turn out to be a mistake, especially if the tendon weakens or ruptures after multiple exposures.

Arthritis expert Joanne Jordan, MD, MPH, Herman and Louise Smith Distinguished Professor of Medicine and director of the Thurston Arthritis Research Center at the University of North Carolina, reminds us that both doctors and patient make a big mistake if they overlook all the nondrug approaches that can be helpful. Weight loss is at the top of her list; getting rid of a few pounds can have a big impact on the knees and other joints. Correcting leg length inequalities with orthotics and utilizing the services of physical therapists is another approach she advocates. She also thinks it is important for patients and doctors to review possible dietary triggers and for the patient's vitamin D level to be checked. Addressing too-low levels of this vitamin can often be surprisingly beneficial in reducing joint pain.[18]

By now it should be clear that there is no nice, neat, one-size-fits-all solution to the problem of alleviating arthritis pain. Products such as glucosamine and chondroitin have been disappointing in double-blind trials.[19] Nonetheless, these supplements don't appear to be dangerous, and many people are convinced that they are helpful.

What may end up working best for arthritis is a combination approach, including physical therapy, topical NSAIDs (or even liniments like capsaicin cream), attention to diet and adequate vitamin D intake, and possibly acupuncture or injection of hyaluronic acid.[20-21] There are plenty of home remedies that people have tried for arthritis, but there is basically no science to tell us whether they are likely to work. Common sense should tell you if there might be a danger in using a remedy you hear about.

ASTHMA

We take breathing for granted. Even though it is possible to hold our breath or take a deep breath voluntarily, most of the time we breathe without paying any attention.

That's not necessarily the case for people with asthma, and there are plenty of them. According to the Centers for Disease Control and Prevention, nearly one child out of ten in this country has asthma,[1] an inflammatory condition that causes chest tightness, a feeling of breathlessness, coughing, and wheezing. Adults, too, may have asthma, though the prevalence is not quite so high. People with asthma may gasp for air during an attack, and sometimes attacks are fatal. When asthma strikes, the lining of the airways swells, reducing the amount of space within for air to move in and out of the lungs. The attack might be triggered by an infection, such as a cold or the flu, or by secondhand smoke, irritating chemicals, or airborne allergens. There is also a hypothesis that some cases of asthma are caused by chronic lung infection.[2]

Some people with asthma have used an over-the-counter inhaler containing epinephrine to overcome wheezing from an occasional attack, or as backup medication if they forget their regular inhaler and start to have an attack. This drug is supposed to provide relief within ten minutes or so, but it is a serious mistake to rely heavily on it. Despite its over-the-counter status, epinephrine can have serious side effects. The Food and Drug Administration will not allow it on the market past December 31, 2011.[3]

Inhaler Danger

"Last January I was rushed to the medical center with a heart attack after taking two puffs from an over-the-counter bronchial mist inhaler. Using the inhaler immediately made me short of breath, and the trauma caused by the reaction caused a heart attack. The doctor told me my life was saved in the emergency room.

"I was hospitalized for three days and the bill came to $23,000. I have no insurance and feel that the pharmacy where I bought the asthma inhaler should pay for my medical bills. I will have to live with a damaged heart for the rest of my life. As an active athlete, this is a considerable price to pay."

Usually, asthma is treated with two different kinds of medications: (1) drugs designed to control inflammation and keep airways from reacting to triggers and (2) drugs designed to open airways during an acute attack. The most common type of anti-inflammatory drug would be an inhaled steroid such as fluticasone (Flovent, also a component of the combination drug Advair) or budesonide (Pulmicort, also a component of the combination drug Symbicort). Within the past decade, an oral medication has been increasingly used to provide ongoing asthma control. Like the inhaled steroids, montelukast (Singulair) pills do not act quickly enough to stop an asthma attack that has begun but instead help to keep inflammation under control so an attack is less likely.

Many people using an inhaled steroid are also given a prescription for a bronchodilator, a drug to open the airways. One such medication is albuterol (ProAir HFA, Proventil, Ventolin). Sometimes the steroid and the bronchodilator are combined in the same inhaler, as salmeterol in the combination drug Advair or formoterol in the combination drug Symbicort. Salmeterol and formoterol are known technically as long-acting beta agonists, or LABAs. These drugs seem to help people with asthma breathe better, and doctors have been pretty enthusiastic about them. Serious questions have been raised about their safety, however.[4] Too many asthma patients have had very severe asthma attacks that required emergency hospitalization or have even died despite using their LABA-containing medication faithfully.[5-7] To try to prevent this, the FDA has recommended that these drugs not be prescribed on their own: *"Use of a LABA alone without use of a long-term asthma control medication, such as an inhaled corticosteroid, is* <u>*contraindicated*</u> *(absolutely advised against) in the treatment of asthma."*[8] Instead, the agency recommends that these drugs be used only in conjunction with inhaled corticosteroids.

According to Dr. Shelley Salpeter, pulmonologists are making a big mistake if they assume that combining the LABAs with corticosteroids totally protects patients from the possible negative effects,[9] and she worries that physicians might become complacent about the dangers of the treatment.[10] Dr. Salpeter's concerns are reinforced by a pilot study showing that children with exercise-induced asthma taking a combo of inhaled steroids and long-acting beta agonists do better when the LABA is discontinued.[11] The Food and Drug Administration has called for new studies to evaluate the safety of LABAs in combination with inhaled corticosteroids. Results may not be available until 2017.

The problem is that doctors have been led to think of these drugs as magic bullets for hard-to-manage asthma. There is no magic bullet, sadly enough. It is not clear that inhaled steroids are as safe as doctors have been told, either. People with chronic obstructive pulmonary disease, a different condition that causes breathing difficulties, treated much the same way asthma is, are at greater risk of pneumonia when they use inhaled steroids long term.[12]

We don't want to sound like therapeutic nihilists. Obviously, people with asthma need help. But there should be a degree of caution and periodic reassessment about the use of the medications. Patients might also want to investigate learning a special breathing technique, called the Buteyko method.[13] Although only a handful of studies have been done on this technique, unlike the thousands of studies of asthma medications, it is an approach that patients themselves control and can evaluate. It may also offer people the chance to work with their doctors to better control a breathing problem.[14] We cannot advocate too strongly that people with asthma must become knowledgeable about their condition and involved in its management.

ATTENTION DEFICIT DISORDER (ADD)

Attention deficit disorder (ADD), with or without hyperactivity, is a trait in which mental focus may wander away from the task at hand. Although there are times when any of us has a hard time staying focused on a boring job, it is even more difficult for those with this trait. With teachers or parents who know how to help children emphasize their strengths and work around their weaknesses, ADD doesn't have to be a huge liability. People with ADD often have great creativity, tenacity, and a strong sense of humor. Nonetheless, ADD can cause trouble for either children or adults with this trait, who might be tempted to fidget, daydream, or bounce around. Adults with ADD may have difficulty holding down a job on a consistent basis, and the condition can contribute to a long-term pattern of underachievement.

There are medications for ADD. These are primarily stimulants, such as methylphenidate (Ritalin) or dextroamphetamine/amphetamine (Adderall), and there has been controversy about the pros and cons of treating of young children with such powerful drugs. For older children and adults, the benefits may be clearer and the risks less worrisome. Making a decision on principle not to use medication to treat ADD could be a big mistake. Many people benefit from one or another drug to help them focus. But the benefit and the need should be reassessed periodically.

One of the most common mistakes made in ADD is assuming there is an objective test that can be administered to determine whether a child has it. There is no blood or urine test for this diagnosis, nor is there a simple five-question list that works. To diagnose ADD properly, an experienced clinician needs input from parents and teachers as well as to observe the child personally. This can be a lengthy process. Many people with ADD are capable of hyperfocusing, especially in a one-on-one setting, so a five-minute interview with the child won't necessarily reveal the problem. The evaluation may take as long as four hours in the hands of an expert like Ned Hallowell, MD (author of *Driven to Distraction* and *Delivered from Distraction*).[1]

Another mistake is to rely exclusively on medication. While these drugs can be very helpful for some people, others don't respond particularly well to them. Behavioral approaches to help children learn how to focus appropriately and channel their energy are now recommended as the first-line treatment for ADD in Great Britain.[2] Parents of children with ADD who answered a *Consumer Reports* survey said the most useful things they did for their children were giving medication (67 percent), changing to a more appropriate school (45 percent), giving instructions one at a time (39 percent), hiring a tutor (37 percent), and providing a consistent schedule (35 percent).[3] These parents also found it essential to advocate for the child, to keep meticulous records, and to assemble a team of experts to help guide the plan for behavioral treatment at home and at school.

Attention to regular exercise, adequate sleep, and a diet that minimizes junk food should always be part of the treatment program, according to Kathi Kemper, MD (author of *Addressing ADD Naturally*).[4] Just exhorting the person with ADD to "try harder" doesn't get to the root of the problem, but coaching for particular behaviors can make a difference. Fish oil at a dose of 2,000 mg daily of combined EPA and DHA (two types of omega-3 fatty acids) can often be helpful, according to Dr. Hallowell.[5] Mindfulness meditation can also be extremely useful in helping a distractible person learn to harness her attention. But if meditation is too much of a challenge for a distractible mind, neurofeedback may offer some promise. The research on this approach is just beginning, though, and the treatment can be costly.[6] For adults, there is fairly good evidence for the benefits of cognitive behavioral therapy, and the gains are maintained over time.[7] Any of these behavioral approaches can be used to bolster treatment with medication.

Simply writing a prescription without making a plan for follow-up is a third mistake. The prescriber needs to monitor how well the medicine works and whether it causes side effects such as stomachache, insomnia, irritability, and slower growth in children or elevated blood pressure in adults. Clinical practice guidelines recommend that this aspect of treatment is equally important as a structured approach to diagnosis in the management of ADD.[8] In practical terms, the patient who has just been diagnosed with ADD or the parent of a child with ADD should not leave the health care provider's office without discussing (1) what behavioral approaches might be helpful and how to get instruction in coaching; (2) how the medicine, if any, should be taken and whether it is needed every day or only on school days; and (3) when the next office visit should be. A person with ADD may have difficulty making a plan for follow-up, so date, time, and other expectations need to be specified right at the outset.

BACK PAIN

Back pain is extraordinarily common. It's so common, in fact, that Nortin Hadler, MD, asserts: "To live a year without a backache is abnormal."[1] In most cases, though, the backache is temporary. It goes away after a few days or weeks, and though it certainly gets our attention while we have it, once it is gone, we forget all about it.

There are backaches that don't go away so quickly, though. And there are times when normal coping strategies don't seem to help as they have in the past. There is evidence that when we are feeling overwhelmed with stress, we have much more difficulty dealing with back pain. But if we take our aching backs to a doctor, there's a pretty good chance that imaging will turn up something that looks a little abnormal to blame for the pain. What the experts tell us is that arthritis in the vertebrae and funny-looking discs between them are fairly standard in most people who are beyond their teenage years. Even though it is tempting to look at the X-ray or other image and decide that the oddity must be responsible for the pain, it is very difficult to prove. Operating on a patient within the first few weeks of regional lower back pain could be quite a screwup, unless there has been trauma and bones are broken.

John Sarno, MD, has explained the difficulty like this: "They [doctors] function more or less like automobile mechanics where the human body is concerned. They are not attuned to psychosomatic phenomena, and that's the problem. And of course that's why they will continue to treat people with physical therapy and with injections and with surgery and the whole kit and caboodle of structural approaches to the problem. You see, attributing this to a structural problem only reinforces the problem. Now the patient says, 'Yeah, I got a bad back. I've got herniated discs back there, but I don't want surgery.' And I'm telling people, 'Your back is normal, but you're hurting because of what's going on in your life.' "[2]

Now, nobody with a backache wants to be told to pull up their socks and get on with their life. What they want is some way to alleviate the pain. Unfortunately, the track record for treatments isn't very good, and the more extreme the treatment, such as surgery, the greater the chance of something going wrong and making matters worse. Dr. Hadler's excellent book *Stabbed in the Back: Confronting Back Pain in an Overtreated Society* presents a thorough overview of the data on treatments for back pain and demonstrates that none is especially effective across the board. Now, before anyone objects that Uncle Charlie got a great deal of relief from a chiropractic manipulation, or an injection, or even a surgical procedure, we just want to specify that these are the data from randomized trials at a population level, not for individual patients. And, indeed, it appears that in most cases, exercising common sense is the safest way to go: don't do things that hurt while the back is hurting, but do resume normal activities when that seems reasonable. These are general guidelines, of course, and each person needs individual evaluation to rule out more serious complications. It should go without saying (but we'll say it anyway) that a person who feels overwhelmed because life seems out of control should muster all the support he or she can manage to address those problems. It will do the sore back a world of good.

BREAST CANCER

Although breast cancer was once a taboo topic, those days are long gone. These days, we are surrounded by pink ribbons; in October, Breast Cancer Awareness Month, it sometimes seems that half the items in the supermarket are swathed in pink. Whether all the public awareness actually contributes to efforts to control breast cancer is, of course, quite another question.

The death rate from breast cancer is approximately 40,000 American women each year, a rate that has decreased by 1.5 to 2 percent per year over the past decade.[1] This cancer is significantly more common among older women than among women under age forty.

There's no shortage of controversy when it comes to diagnosing and treating breast cancer. Take the best age at which to begin screening mammography and the appropriate intervals for this "early detection" test, for example. When a careful analysis of screening mammography and mortality noted that screening women between the ages of fifty and sixty-nine every two years provided the best reduction in breast cancer deaths with the least harm,[2] there was quite an outcry. The U.S. Preventive Services Task Force recommended in November 2009 that women between ages forty and forty-nine should not undergo routine annual screening mammograms and was promptly criticized by some patients and by groups such as the American Cancer Society and the American College of Radiology.[3] There was much less uproar about its recommendation that women older than seventy-four stop getting routine screening mammography. The controversy may not go away for some time. Swedish scientists announced, a year after the Task Force recommendation, that their analysis vindicated screening women under age fifty.[4] In a nationwide study, they found that mammography reduced breast cancer mortality in this younger age group.

The problem with screening women under age forty is that cumulative radiation from the mammogram itself may increase the risk of cancer. Experts also worry about the harms women may suffer if a mammogram incorrectly identifies a potential cancer and the woman then is put through an unnecessary biopsy and perhaps further testing, not to mention the worry. Receiving a diagnosis of breast cancer is practically guaranteed to create enormous anxiety, even if it later turns out to have been a false alarm.

We spoke with breast cancer expert Dr. Susan Love, president of the Dr. Susan Love Research Foundation, about how women can avoid mistakes when it comes to breast cancer.[5] She points out that mammograms are not perfect: in addition to the tests that wrongly finger apparent but nonexistent breast tumors, there are mammograms that fail to detect breast cancers that are present, giving the woman a false sense of security.

Not every cancer that is detected deserves treatment. Just as with prostate cancer, there are some breast tumors that do not progress, especially those termed ductal carcinoma in situ (DCIS). Treating these cancers aggressively may be a mistake, since only about one-third of them progress to become invasive; unfortunately, it is not possible to tell the difference between cancers that are just going to sit there quietly for the rest of a woman's life and those that are going to cause trouble. This complicates decision-making enormously.

The average woman who is diagnosed with cancer in one breast and does not have a genetic risk might make a mistake if she decides to have the other breast removed as a preventive measure. Dr. Love likens that to trying to appease mysterious gods, or perhaps to slamming the barn door after the horse has already fled. She points out two things: first, that breast cancer in the opposite breast is not really very common, although it certainly does happen; and second, that even with mastectomy, it is possible (though again, not common) to get a recurrence in the scar. She advocates that women look at all of their options carefully before rushing to have this surgery. For the woman with a BRCA gene that puts her at very high risk, of course, the calculation is different. Preventive mastectomy and even removal of the ovaries, though extreme, does offer such women a measure of protection.[6] A meta-analysis of all the studies that had been done on this issue came to the same conclusions, that removing the noncancerous breast preventively does not seem to improve survival, and that prophylactic mastectomy of both breasts should be reserved for women at extremely high risk of the disease.[7]

CELIAC DISEASE

People with celiac disease are exquisitely sensitive to gluten, a protein found in wheat, barley, and rye. A component of this protein, gliadin, triggers an autoimmune response in the bodies of such people, starting in the small intestine. The lining of the intestine becomes smoother and less capable of absorbing a wide range of nutrients. That in itself contributes to many of the long-term complications of celiac disease, such as neurological damage due to vitamin B_{12} malabsorption or osteoporosis due to poor absorption of minerals.[1] The immune system's attack on the body reaches beyond the digestive tract, however, and may also affect the nervous system.[2-3]

Probably the biggest screwup when it comes to celiac disease is overlooking the diagnosis. At one time, doctors were taught that celiac disease was extremely rare, affecting only about 1 in 5,000 people.[4] As a result, patients who complained of nonspecific symptoms such as weakness, tiredness, headaches, abdominal pain, chronic canker sores, or anemia might not be worked up for celiac disease. Sometimes it took years for a patient to discover that celiac disease was at the root of all these troubles.

In recent years, it has become clear that celiac disease is far more common, affecting approximately 1 percent of the population in Europe[5] and just slightly less than that in the United States, though it has increased since 1974.[6] When one person in the family has been diagnosed with celiac disease, there is a much higher chance that others will have it as well, perhaps as high as one in five.[7] The correct procedure for diagnosis has generated a certain amount of controversy.[8] As we have seen, the symptoms can be somewhat nonspecific; the gold standard has been microscopic examination of a biopsy of the small intestine showing changes in the lining. Not surprisingly, relatively few people are enthusiastic about this procedure, so when they learn there are blood tests for the diagnosis, they are much more willing to be tested. These are tests for tissue transglutaminase (TTG) and endomysial (EMA) antibodies, and they are very helpful in making the diagnosis.[9] But many doctors are not aware that none of these tests is totally accurate by itself, not even the biopsy.[10] Instead, experts now recommend a "four-out-of-five" approach to diagnosing: symptoms typical of celiac disease; positive blood tests; positive genotype test for the genetic markers for celiac disease, HLA-DQ2 or HLA-DQ8; typical celiac pathological changes in the bowel biopsy; and improvement on a gluten-free diet.[11]

One possible screwup that patients may be tempted to make is self-diagnosis and self-treatment with a gluten-free diet. Although it is true that this is the recommended treatment for celiac disease, embarking on the gluten-free diet prior to medical diagnosis can make a diagnosis even more difficult. What's more, symptomatic improvement on a gluten-free diet doesn't necessarily mean that a person has celiac disease.[12] However, there's nothing wrong with a person's deciding to avoid gluten because she feels better without it, though such a diet may pose a challenge.

A person who has celiac disease must be absolutely fastidious about avoiding all gluten because of the danger of complications of the celiac disease resulting from exposure to gluten. The most frightening of these complications is cancer.[13] For the celiac disease sufferer, following a gluten-free diet is actually a matter of life and death, even though it is very challenging. Taking a laissez-faire approach would be a major patient screwup. That is why doctors treating patients they have di-agnosed with celiac disease are urged to connect their patients with advocacy groups such as the Celiac Disease Foundation (www.celiac .org) or www.celiac.com. Such sites often offer recipes and guidance on achieving a palatable gluten-free diet. Though it will require a great deal of diligence, a gluten-free diet is the only treatment for celiac disease at this time, and it is absolutely essential.

DEEP VEIN THROMBOSIS (DVT)

When a blood clot lodges in a coronary artery, it's called a heart attack. In the brain, a similar event is called a stroke. In both cases, the symp-toms often come on fairly quickly, and doctors have strategies for fast diagnosis. When a blood clot forms in a vein rather than an artery, the symptoms can be subtle and harder to assess. Perhaps that is why deep vein thrombosis (DVT) and its consequences (pulmonary embolism, or a blood clot in the lungs) are often misdiagnosed and are a leading cause of malpractice lawsuits.[1-3] The Centers for Disease Control and Prevention estimate that anywhere from 300,000 to 600,000 people experience a DVT or a pulmonary embolism in any given year.[4] Other researchers put the number much higher—anywhere from 900,000 to 1 million serious venous blood clots annually.[5-6] As many as 300,000 people die annually as a result of such blood clots.[7]

When someone develops a blood clot in a vein in the legs, the symp-toms can be somewhat vague. There may be a sense of tightness in the leg or it may feel a little like a leg cramp. Since these may be perceived as seemingly unimportant signs, neither the patient nor the physician may take them very seriously at first. But if a blood clot breaks loose from the legs and lodges in the lungs, it can cause sudden death, though here, too, symptoms can sometimes be subtle initially—shortness of breath, cough, or generalized chest pain.

To better understand the problems surrounding DVT and its complications we interviewed Thomas Ortel, MD, PhD.[8] He is one of the country's leading experts on these issues and coauthor of *100 Questions and Answers About Deep Vein Thrombosis and Pulmonary Embolism*. We asked Dr. Ortel about common mistakes, and he replied: "Frequently, the most common mistake is just simply missing the diagnosis. And it's because many patients may have other problems affecting the limbs. They may have edema [fluid buildup] from heart failure or other problems and so the symptoms may not be noticed or carefully distinguished, or somebody may overlook it, or patients may underplay it or may not complain as much as they should to be sure they are being evaluated carefully and completely enough. So it can be missed." When Dr. Ortel presents to the medical students, he sometimes brings a patient who had a hard time getting a correct diagnosis. She had wrenched her knee at the beach, and that was all her doctors could focus on. In addition to the knee injury, she also had a blood clot. Even though she came back time after time complaining about her discomfort, the DVT was missed because her doctors were concentrating on the knee problem.

Patients must be assertive when it comes to a potential diagnosis of DVT or pulmonary embolism. If there is pain, tenderness, swelling, redness, or a feeling of heat in one leg (or arm), medical attention is required. (It would be rare for both legs or both arms to have a clot simultaneously.) A diffuse reddish or bluish skin discoloration would also be a symptom to look for. When you get to the emergency department, ask to be evaluated for a DVT with an ultrasound machine. Symptoms of a pulmonary embolism include sudden shortness of breath, chest pain that may worsen with deep breathing, and/or a cough that can't be explained by a cold. A CT (computerized tomography) or an MRI (magnetic resonance imaging) can help diagnose a blood clot in the lungs. A great resource for patients is the National Blood Clot Alliance. For more information and resources visit www.stoptheclot.org.

DEPRESSION

There was a time when patients who complained about feeling depressed were referred to an expert—a psychiatrist, a psychologist, or a psychiatric social worker. They would be carefully evaluated, and a treatment plan would be considered that might involve talking therapy (psychotherapy or some other form of counseling). Sometimes an antidepressant would be prescribed. The benefits and side effects of the medication could be tracked during weekly therapy sessions.

These days, everyone is in a hurry. Patients want a quick fix, insurance companies are not thrilled with the idea of paying for months of therapy, and primary care doctors have become convinced that they can treat depression as well as specialists, and often that involves a prescription for an antidepressant. Such medications are among the most widely prescribed drugs in the United States.[1] At last count, over 160 million prescriptions were dispensed for pharmaceuticals such as bupropion (Wellbutrin), citalopram (Celexa), desvenlafaxine (Pristiq), duloxetine (Cymbalta), escitalopram (Lexapro), fluoxetine (Prozac), paroxetine (Paxil), sertraline (Zoloft), and venlafaxine (Effexor). The most likely explanation for so many antidepressant prescriptions is that nurse practitioners, family practice physicians, internists, and many other physicians are prescribing antidepressants for a wide range of psychological symptoms.

The only problem with this picture is that it relies so heavily on pharmacotherapy alone and does not take into consideration many other approaches. We also wonder whether most of these prescribers have taken the time to read the scientific literature about the actual effectiveness of antidepressants for treating mild to moderate psychological depression. If they had, we doubt these drugs would be prescribed in such quantity.

In 2010, a meta-analysis of high-quality antidepressant clinical trials from January 1980 through March 2009 was published in the *Journal of the American Medical Association.*[2] The investigators concluded that such drugs help people with long-lasting "very severe symptoms." But most of the prescriptions for antidepressants are written for individuals with mild to moderate depression. In this population, there is little evidence that antidepressants are helpful. In the words of the researchers: "True drug effects (an advantage of ADM [antidepressant medication] over placebo) were nonexistent to negligible among depressed patients with mild, moderate, and even severe baseline symptoms."[3]

This is not the first study to throw doubt on the value of antidepressants for mild or moderate depression. In 2008, Irving Kirsch, MD, and his colleagues reported that highly successful antidepressants such as Celexa, Effexor, Paxil, Prozac, Serzone, and Zoloft hardly worked better than placebos in clinical trials.[4] A cover story in *Newsweek* summed it up this way: "As more and more scientists who study depression and the drugs that treat it are concluding, that suggests that antidepressants are basically expensive Tic Tacs."[5]

Antidepressant Disappointment

"For about 85 percent of the patients who are clinically depressed who take these drugs, the drug will not outperform a placebo, and that is absolutely stunning. It's a breathtaking finding, and it's one that should give us all pause in the field."[6]

Clinical psychologist Stephen Ilardi, PhD, May 29, 2010

We suspect that relatively few primary care providers bother to read the official prescribing information found with popular antidepressants, which states specifically that they are "indicated for the acute maintenance treatment of major depressive disorder. . . . A major depressive episode (DSM-IV) implies a prominent and relatively persistent (nearly every day for at least 2 weeks) depressed or dysphoric mood that usually interferes with daily functioning, and includes at least 5 of the following 9 symptoms: depressed mood, loss of interest in usual activities, significant change in weight and/or appetite, insomnia or hypersomnia, psychomotor agitation or retardation, increased fatigue, feelings of guilt or worthlessness, slowed thinking or impaired concentration, or a suicide attempt or suicidal ideation." If a prescriber is unaware that antidepressants have been approved by the Food and Drug Administration (FDA) for *only* "major depression," that is a serious screwup. Failing to warn patients and families that antidepressants may increase the risk of suicidal thoughts and behaviors would be another.

Suicide Warning

"Patients of all ages who are started on antidepressant therapy should be monitored appropriately and observed closely for clinical worsening, suicidality, or unusual changes in behavior. Families and caregivers should be advised of the need for close observation and communication with the prescriber."

Official FDA black-box warning

Some physicians may also forget to mention that stopping many antidepressants suddenly can lead to unpleasant withdrawal symptoms. They can include dizziness, nausea, headaches, nervousness, insomnia, sweating, shakiness, visual disturbances, weakness, and difficulty concentrating. Many people also report electric shock–like sensations. Some describe this as "brain shivers." Since drug companies rarely provide guidelines about how to *stop* their medications, prescribers have to make this up as they go. As a result, many physicians do not have a clue as to how someone should phase off an antidepressant. We consider this a significant screwup.

If antidepressants don't represent a lasting cure for most individuals with mild to moderate depression, what else is available? A lifestyle approach might be far more effective than many physicians realize. Stephen Ilardi, PhD, is a researcher and clinical psychologist with twenty years of experience. He believes that the way we live our lives makes a huge difference in our mental health. In reviewing the literature and working with patients, he has identified successful strategies to help people deal with depression without drugs. His six steps include: physical exercise, dietary omega-3 fatty acids (found in fish oil), engaging activity that prevents rumination (brooding or dwelling on negative thoughts), sunlight exposure, social support, and sleep. By combining all of these elements together, he has achieved a substantially greater improvement in depressed patients than standard therapy with antidepressant medications.[7] Of course, this kind of approach requires time and coaching. We wish more physicians would consider Dr. Ilardi's approach (found in his book *The Depression Cure*) along with psychotherapy instead of quickly writing a prescription for an antidepressant medication that might not be better than placebo.

DIABETES

Type 2 diabetes has become one of the world's most worrisome health problems. In the United States, the statistics are truly overwhelming. If one believes the American Diabetes Association (ADA), there are nearly 24 million citizens with diabetes, roughly one-third of whom are undiagnosed.[1] If you think the numbers from the ADA are scary, consider the projections from the Centers for Disease Control and Prevention. These federal folks have no particular ax to grind. They state that "as many as 1 in 3 U.S. adults could have diabetes by 2050 if current trends continue."[2] Compare that to 1 in 10 today.

But it gets worse. According to the ADA number crunchers, there are almost 60 million people with something categorized as prediabetes. People with this condition have blood glucose numbers that are elevated but not yet high enough to be diagnosed with frank diabetes. Chances are that many of these individuals are carrying extra pounds, especially distributed around the midsection, and they may also have high triglyceride levels in the blood. This prediabetic state has much in common with something called metabolic syndrome, which is characterized by "abdominal adiposity" (big belly), high triglycerides, and low

HDL (high-density lipoprotein) cholesterol, insulin resistance (the body doesn't utilize insulin properly), and high c-reactive protein levels in the blood (a measurement of inflammation in the body).[3] Prediabetics are at increased risk for type 2 diabetes, heart attacks, strokes, and other cardiovascular complications. If you lump people with diabetes and prediabetes together and look just a decade ahead, half of all Americans could be affected.[4]

What's causing this incredible epidemic? Unless you have been living in a cave, you have heard that much of the blame rests on eating too much and exercising too little. That's what the experts repeat like a mantra, and we won't disagree. All one has to do is look around to see that an astonishing number of Americans are overweight and out of shape. That said, there could also be environmental factors that are contributing to the diabetes disaster. Pesticides, organic pollutants like PCBs (polychlorinated biphenyls), dioxins, mercury, bisphenol-A (BPA), and phthalates (found in many flexible plastic products) are just some of the compounds that may affect insulin resistance.[5-10] There is also growing concern that high fructose corn syrup, which is found in many beverages as a sweetener, might increase the risk of insulin resistance.[11-13] We think it is a screwup that medicine has not paid more attention to these environmental factors as it bemoans the diabetes epidemic.

What about diet? If ever there has been a screwup in the prevention and management of diabetes, it has to be centered around diet. For decades, experts have been arguing about the best diet to help control blood sugar. Twenty years ago, we asked leading diabetologists whether eating a lot of sugar and sweetened foods would increase a person's risk of developing type 2 diabetes. Back then, we were told categorically no.

More recently, though, carbohydrates, particularly refined or highly processed carbs, have come under scrutiny. High-glycemic-index foods cause a quick rise in blood sugar and insulin. These are things like sugar, white bread, and potatoes. Chips, candy, pretzels, pizza, soft drinks, juice, and french fries would be examples of high-glycemic-index snacks. Low-glycemic index foods such as lentils or fish do not cause the rapid rise in blood sugar. Despite this, the American Diabetes Association has held the position that there is not sufficient evidence that diets low in glycemic load help prevent diabetes.

Research from the Netherlands suggests, however, that such evidence is becoming available. A large study of more than 37,000 people followed for an average of ten years found that high-glycemic-load diets were associated with a greater risk of developing type 2 diabetes. The authors concluded that "both carbohydrate quantity and quality seem to be important factors in diabetes prevention."[14] There is growing awareness that the degree of blood sugar elevation following food is an important factor in the development of diabetes and other chronic diseases.[15]

When Richard Bernstein, MD, first published his book *Dr. Bernstein's Diabetes Solution* in 1997, the medical establishment and the American Diabetes Association reacted as if he were on the fringe. Dr. Bernstein developed his approach from his own experience.[16] He was diagnosed with type 1 diabetes at age twelve. As an engineer and the spouse of a physician, he was fascinated with an emerging technology to measure blood sugar and acquired one of the earliest devices for his own use. Experimentation with his diet revealed that avoiding easily digested starches and sugars allowed him to control his blood sugar much better than before.

At age forty-five, Richard Bernstein started medical school, partly so that he could disseminate these findings and help other people with diabetes. He was so far ahead of his time, however, that his message has had an uphill struggle. Historically, both the American Heart Association and the American Diabetes Association focused more on avoiding fat than on cautioning against carbohydrates. Dr. Bernstein's research suggested that carbs were a bigger problem in blood sugar control.

Experts have known for years that many people with type 2 diabetes can often be controlled without drugs, so long as the patient is conscientious about exercise and diet. Many of the doctors who treat diabetes are pessimistic that their patients will actually be diligent enough, but perhaps that is because of the diet advice screwup. Even now, many doctors who treat people with diabetes are not convinced that it makes sense for their patients to learn about glycemic index and glycemic load. But there are research-based resources that can be very helpful.[17-18] Generally, people with diabetes want to keep these high GI foods out of their diet and eat more foods with a lower glycemic index. We think *Dr. Bernstein's Diabetes Solution* provides a helpful approach to achieving better blood sugar control, even if mainstream medicine has still not embraced his perspective. For information on the glycemic index of specific foods, the following website can be helpful: www .glycemicindex.com.

Few physicians have been trained how to coach patients to maintain healthy eating and exercise programs. As a result, doctors often feel frustrated when people with diabetes don't lose weight or control blood sugar adequately. The consequence is that many physicians rely on drugs to do the job. We don't want to downplay the importance of medications. They can work very well to bring elevated blood glucose levels into the normal range. But there has been an earthquake within the world of diabetes care, and many experts are having a hard time dealing with the aftermath.

For years, physicians have played a numbers game when it comes to treating people with diabetes. Because people with this disease are more likely to experience heart attacks, strokes, kidney disease, loss of circulation to the legs and feet, nerve damage, vision loss, and cognitive impairment, experts have come up with guidelines to keep blood sugar, cholesterol, and blood pressure as close to normal as possible. To reach the target range, it is not unusual for physicians to prescribe multiple medications, all with the hope of preventing the complications of diabetes.

The trouble with this approach, however, is that aggressive control of blood sugar, blood pressure, and blood fats does not keep people with diabetes from dying prematurely of heart attacks and strokes.[19-23] In fact, patients under intensive treatment to lower blood sugar actually fared worse and died sooner than those who experienced less aggressive control.[24] It turns out that if blood sugar levels fall too low, it can be just as risky as if they climb too high. A huge study called ACCORD (which stands for Action to Control Cardiovascular Risk in Diabetes) included thousands of patients over several years and was supposed to demonstrate that "tight control" with drugs would be superior to less stringent efforts. It didn't work out that way. The results of ACCORD shook the medical community to its core. At the time of this writing, many diabetes experts are still shaking their heads in amazement about the unexpected and disappointing outcome of the ACCORD trial.

Another diabetes treatment screwup involved the drug rosiglitazone (Avandia), one of the most successful diabetes drugs of all time. In 2006, over 11.3 million prescriptions were dispensed, and the drug garnered sales of over $3 billion.[25] Avandia worked quite well to control blood sugar levels. There was only one problem. This drug did not improve outcomes that really mattered—a reduction in heart attacks and strokes. If anything, Avandia increased the risk of cardiovascular complications.[26] Eventually, European regulators banned Avandia, and the U.S. Food and Drug Administration severely restricted its use.

Many physicians may have assumed that Avandia was an anomaly. There was, however, a far more fundamental lesson to be learned from this experience. Just lowering blood glucose does not guarantee improvement in the things that really matter—fewer heart attacks and strokes, less kidney damage, and improved overall mortality statistics.

Over forty years ago, a huge government-sponsored study (UGDP [University Group Diabetes Program]) also shocked the medical community. It turned out that people treated with the oral diabetes drug tolbutamide (Orinase) were more likely to have heart attacks, related heart problems, and more deaths than patients treated by diet alone or with insulin.[27] Physicians argued about the significance of the data for years. Finally, a careful analysis concluded that the results were accurate and cautioned that proponents of oral diabetes drugs had to "conduct scientifically adequate studies to justify continued use of such agents."[28]

Decades later, though, we still lack long-term studies proving that most oral diabetes drugs do anything more than lower blood sugar. That's necessary, but not sufficient. What patients with diabetes deserve are medications that not only improve results on a blood sugar test but lower their risk of experiencing heart attacks, strokes, nerve damage, kidney failure, blindness, and all the other complications of this disease. Such drugs should also improve mortality statistics. Until that is demonstrated, patients will need a lot of support eating the proper foods and exercising to their ability. And physicians will need to be very thoughtful when it comes to prescribing the best medicine for any particular patient. Most important, our favorite diabetes expert, John Buse, MD, PhD, wants people with diabetes to be diagnosed early to prevent complications. (Dr. Buse is Professor of Medicine and Chief of Endocrinology at the University of North Carolina at Chapel Hill and director of the Diabetes Care Center there. He is also a past president of the American Diabetes Association.) Dr. Buse encourages patients to stay positive, stay focused, and believe that they can control their disease. He points out that people don't have to be perfect, just be better than they were a year ago.

FIBROMYALGIA

Fibromyalgia is the name given to a syndrome in which a person develops a set of symptoms that don't seem to be rooted in structural changes or inflammation. The syndrome entails widespread long-lasting pain in muscles and other soft tissues, especially at specific tender trigger points, along with sleep disturbances, fatigue, problems with other pain such as irritable bowel syndrome or chronic headaches, and even brain "fuzziness." Morning stiffness, tingling and numbness, depression, and anxiety are other problems that frequently accompany the syndrome.[1] According to the National Fibromyalgia Association, as many as 10 million Americans may suffer from fibromyalgia, with women afflicted far more frequently than men.[2]

Fibromyalgia was an extremely controversial topic for many years. The fact that most of the tests a doctor would run on a patient generally give results within the normal range led some doctors to assume that this syndrome is a manifestation of depression or some other type of psychosomatic disorder. Evidence has been accumulating to suggest that people with fibromyalgia are exceptionally sensitive to pain caused by pressure, heat, cold, or other stimuli.[3] One doctor who has specialized in treating people with fibromyalgia, Jacob Teitelbaum, MD, medical director of the Fibromyalgia and Fatigue Centers, suggests that the biggest mistake physicians make when treating fibromyalgia is not recognizing what they don't know. Dr. Teitelbaum told us, "Doctors say to the patient, 'I don't know what this is, so you must be crazy.'"[4] He continued by stating that people do best if they go to doctors who have experience and success in treating this condition.

The doctors who conclude that there is a psychological component are not entirely mistaken. Fibromyalgia is clearly a mind-body disorder. The current understanding is that a range of factors, including stress, mood, and behavior, combine to create changes in hormones, neurotransmitters, and the immune system that alter the way the nervous system responds to pain,[5] referred to as "central sensitization."[6] As a result of this complex causative chain, it doesn't make sense to narrow treatment to a single focus such as drugs. The medications that have been approved by the Food and Drug Administration for the treatment of fibromyalgia can be helpful, but none is a "silver bullet."[7-8] Duloxetine (Cymbalta), milnacipran (Savella), and pregabalin (Lyrica) all have potentially serious side effects, including a potential for suicidal preoccupation, and a wide range of other medications with which they might interact. None of these drugs should be stopped suddenly but rather must be tapered off gradually to avoid unpleasant withdrawal symptoms. People with fibromyalgia appear to do best when nondrug approaches are integrated into their treatment along with medication.[9-11] Generally, the treatment plan should be individualized for each patient. Cognitive-behavioral counseling and graduated exercise programs seem to be among the most effective nondrug therapies.[12-13]

People with fibromyalgia have a great deal of difficulty getting restful sleep. As a result, physicians may prescribe benzodiazepines as sleeping pills. This is a mistake, according to Dr. Teitelbaum, as is the use of NSAID (nonsteroidal anti-inflammatory drug) pain relievers such as ibuprofen (Advil, Motrin, etc.) or naproxen (Aleve) for the trigger-point pain. Those medications do not work as well for fibromyalgia symptoms as doctors might anticipate, and chronic use can lead to trouble. NSAIDs, as we have discussed elsewhere, can lead to serious digestive complications, including bleeding ulcers. Benzodiazepines such as alprazolam (Niravam, Xanax), clonazepam (Klonopin), diazepam (Valium), or lorazepam (Ativan) may lead to dependence if used on a regular basis. Stopping such a drug suddenly after long-term use is an error that can set off uncomfortable withdrawal symptoms.

Because the predominant symptoms of fibromyalgia are muscle pain and fatigue, it is hardly surprising that sometimes people who suffer from this condition make the big mistake of avoiding exercise. Although jumping headfirst into a rigorous training program is hardly advised and might make matters worse, quite a bit of recent research supports the benefits of gentle exercise such as tai chi[14] or yoga[15] in easing fibromyalgia symptoms. An analysis of thirty-four clinical trials found evidence that supervised aerobic exercise is beneficial.[16] The supplement D-ribose was found to be helpful in a small preliminary study,[17] but alternative therapies in general have not been strikingly successful.[18] Stress management and learning to pace activity throughout the day are important strategies for the person with fibromyalgia to master so that symptoms will be less disruptive.

HEARTBURN

Heartburn, or acid reflux, is a truly unpleasant sensation of burning that starts beneath the breastbone and rises toward the throat. As the name suggests, it is presumably caused by acid escaping from the stomach, where it is created and needed for digestion, into the lower esophagus, or swallowing tube. This happens presumably because the ring of muscle at the bottom of the esophagus relaxes inappropriately and opens to let the stomach juices out. It is a surprisingly common problem. As many as 40 percent of Americans may experience heartburn occasionally, while about 20 percent have a severe or chronic condition.

One big problem that interferes with appropriate treatment is a lack of communication.[1] People are not necessarily comfortable talking about embarrassing digestive symptoms. But for your doctor to make a good diagnosis, she'll need a fairly clear description of how you feel: when does the symptom occur, how long does it last, what kind of discomfort is it, and where does it bother you? If it wakes you at night, that is also important information, since reflux is sometimes the cause of chronic insomnia.[2] It is important for the doctor to learn if you are having reflux several times a week, not only so that you can improve your quality of life, but also so that your lower esophagus does not develop abnormal cells (Barrett's esophagus) that could eventually go on to become cancerous. Esophageal cancer is difficult to treat, so here is a situation where an ounce of prevention is definitely worth a pound of cure!

One major screwup that people sometimes make is to assume that the pain in their chests is "just heartburn." It may be nothing more than heartburn, but severe chest pain, particularly if it is different from previous episodes of heartburn or connected to other symptoms such as pain down the left arm or up to the jaw or a sensation of pressure, should be treated as a medical emergency. If this happens to you, call 911 so you can be evaluated for a possible heart attack.

Doctors sometimes give their heartburn patients a long list of foods to avoid, including fried food, mint, tomatoes, chocolate, coffee, tea, alcohol, or spicy food. There's nothing wrong with experimenting to see if any of these forbidden foods actually triggers your reflux symptoms, but there is a surprising lack of evidence to support these recommendations. Physicians sometimes fail to mention a couple of habits that could alleviate heartburn. One is as simple as chewing gum. Chewing on a piece of sugarless gum after a meal can stimulate saliva production, and saliva washes acid back down from the esophagus into the stomach.[3]

The other habit that physicians should recommend is also simple, but far from easy. Doctors know that extra pounds make reflux worse, but they don't always recommend that their patients lose weight. In some cases, this can make a huge difference, even when the weight loss is modest. There is also evidence that a low-carb diet can relieve symptoms even before the person is successful at losing a lot of weight.[4] Too often a doctor commits an oversight by not recommending a trial of a low-carb diet similar to Atkins or South Beach diets to see if it will help the patient with heartburn symptoms in the short run and with weight loss in the longer term.

In fact, the usual recommendation is medication with a class of drugs known as proton pump inhibitors (PPIs). Medicines such as rabeprazole (Aciphex), esomeprazole (Nexium), lansoprazole (Prevacid), omeprazole (Prilosec), or pantoprazole (Protonix) are quite effective in shutting down excess acid secretion, and they can be very useful in helping to ease heartburn symptoms. The problem is that they are so effective that both doctors and patients might be tempted to overuse them. (Prevacid, also sold as lansoprazole; Prilosec, its generic omeprazole; and a combination drug, Zegerid, are available without a prescription.)

Long-term use of PPIs could lead to a number of complications.[5] Some research suggests that people who take one of these drugs for several years are at increased risk of osteoporosis and bone fracture.[6-7] Other studies have shown that people taking one of these drugs for extended periods of time are more susceptible to pneumonia,[8-9] although not all investigators agree.[10] There is also evidence that people on acid-suppressing drugs long-term are at higher risk of catching *Clostridium difficile,* an intestinal infection that can cause devastating diarrhea.[11] Vitamin B_{12} requires an acid environment in the stomach for proper absorption, so some people who take a PPI for many months or years may be at risk of vitamin B_{12} deficiency.[12]

One reason that people may take one of these drugs for a long time is that it can be difficult to stop. A Danish study demonstrated the problem by giving esomeprazole or a placebo to healthy volunteers who had no symptoms of reflux at the beginning of the study.[13] After two months on esomeprazole, the subjects in the intervention group were given a placebo without their knowledge, and they experienced heartburn symptoms for the next month as a result of acid rebound from discontinuing the acid suppressor. Unless the doctor is prepared to help a patient through the process of weaning off a PPI, a person might keep on taking it for years. In the past, doctors assumed that symptoms that cropped up when the drug was stopped meant that the patient still had symptomatic heartburn and still required treatment. We now believe that is a screwup that requires reevaluation.

One last caution regarding PPIs affects people with heart problems who have had a stent placed in a coronary artery to keep it open. Many stents now are coated with a medication that prevents arterial tissue from growing back and "clogging the line," so to speak. But the best practice with such stents is for the patient to take an anticlotting drug called clopidogrel (Plavix) for at least a year after stent placement. This medication can lead to ulcers and intestinal bleeding, but an acid-suppressing drug given to protect the digestive tract may interact with the clopidogrel and make it less effective.[14] This interaction is quite controversial, with some researchers questioning its importance[15-16] while others warn that PPIs are associated with a greater risk for cardiovascular complications after a heart attack regardless of whether or not the patient is taking clopidogrel.[17]

The bottom line is that people who want to avoid screwups in treating their heartburn need to find out what they can do themselves and work closely with their physicians. It makes a lot of sense to get a clear understanding of both the benefits and the risks of the medicines that are being prescribed. Before starting on an acid suppressor, a person should ask about its potential interactions and how long it should be taken and should also get a plan for discontinuing it when the time is right.

HYPOTHYROIDISM

Hypothyroidism is a long word to describe a little gland not working as well as it should. The term simply means "low thyroid function," and since the function of the thyroid gland is to produce thyroid hormone, anyone with too little thyroid hormone circulating in the bloodstream is hypothyroid. As many as 10 million Americans may fall into this category.[1]

People with underactive thyroid glands are often relieved to get a diagnosis that accounts for all the symptoms that have been plaguing them. Some of the more common symptoms include fatigue, weakness, dry skin, brittle hair and fingernails, as well as hair loss. Losing the outer third of the eyebrows is especially indicative of low thyroid function. Hypothyroid people are often especially sensitive to cold, and women may have heavy menstrual periods and difficulty conceiving. The pulse may be slow, and exercise may bring on shortness of breath. Blood tests show anemia and high cholesterol. Weight loss is usually a challenge, but it is even more difficult for those with too little thyroid activity. Possibly the worst symptoms are the most subjective ones because the person may not connect them to a medical condition: apathy, clumsiness, mental slowness, and depression. It is not unusual for a person with too little thyroid hormone to be diagnosed initially as depressed and put on an antidepressant. When this happens, not only is the proper treatment delayed, but antidepressants such as fluoxetine (Prozac), paroxetine (Paxil), or sertraline (Zoloft) have on rare occasions been linked to thyroid disruption.

Diagnostic Delay

"I was diagnosed with 'depression,' and for several years I took a series of different antidepressant drugs. The results were unsatisfactory, and I experienced many unpleasant side effects.

"Then one year I was hospitalized for an unrelated medical problem. During the tests, I was found to be suffering from severe hypothyroidism. I needed Synthroid, not Zoloft!"

Mary Shomon maintains two websites that supply information about thyroid dysfunction and has written a number of books on the topic, including *Living Well with Hypothyroidism.*[2] When we asked her about the top screwups in the treatment of hypothyroidism, she listed a refusal to test for thyroid function in the first place.[3] Many people have reported to us that it took several medical visits, sometimes to more than one doctor, before blood was drawn for a test of thyroid function.

Another mess-up also pertains to diagnosis: paying more attention to the number on the blood test than to the patient's symptoms can also delay the diagnosis. Ms. Shomon called this "slavish dedication to the TSH test to the exclusion of practicing medicine." She observed that sometimes, if the lab result for TSH (thyroid-stimulating hormone) is on the borderline, even though the patient has a lot of very typical symptoms, there are doctors who will not treat for a thyroid problem. They adhere to the "tyranny of the TSH" even though there is considerable controversy among specialists as to just where the normal range of TSH should cut off.[4-5] Specialists also disagree about the value of treating patients within the questionable range of TSH.[6-7]

What is TSH and why should it matter? TSH, thyroid-stimulating hormone, is part of the wonderful feedback system our bodies use to make sure that the glands are working normally. TSH works a bit like a thermostat for the thyroid; when the brain senses that there is not enough active thyroid hormone circulating in the bloodstream, it sends a message to the thyroid gland to step up its activity. That messenger, thyroid-stimulating hormone, stimulates the thyroid gland to make more. That makes TSH a pretty sensitive, but upside-down, measure of how well the thyroid gland is working. When TSH is normal, there's usually enough thyroxine (thyroid hormone). But if TSH is high, that indicates not enough thyroxine. (There are some situations in which this relationship falls apart, such as when the pituitary gland in the brain isn't working properly and is the source of the problem. Failure to investigate that would be another type of error.)

TSH is measured through a blood test, and the doctor can test for circulating thyroid hormones (T_3 and T_4) at the same time. As mentioned, doctors disagree about whether the cutoff for normal TSH should be at 3.5 or at 5 mIU/L (milli–international units per liter). But they are also arguing among themselves about whether or not to treat "subclinical" hypothyroidism.[8-10] As defined by the specialists, subclinical hypothyroidism is when the TSH is above normal, but thyroxine, aka T_4, the main thyroid hormone, is within the normal range, regardless of whether the patient has symptoms. Of course, to us it seems that the person's symptoms would be relevant and that *subclinical* would refer to a person with none. But not in number-conscious medical practice.

Why should hypothyroidism be treated? There are two reasons. The most important is that treatment generally helps the patient feel better. Quality of life is important, and people with symptoms of underactive thyroid are not enjoying the best quality of life. The other reason is that untreated thyroid disease is thought to have an impact on cardiovascular risk. Whether that is because of the elevated cholesterol associated with low thyroxine or because of other factors, it makes sense to reduce heart disease risk when it is practical.

Mary Shomon suggested one other mistake, which is to offer patients only one treatment option. Generally, doctors prefer to prescribe levothyroxine (T_4, also available as the brand names Levothroid, Levoxyl, and Synthroid). This synthetic hormone works well as a replacement for many hypothyroid people, but not for everyone. Some people seem to do better on therapies that combine T_3 (triiodothyronine) with T_4. And this is the subject of significant controversy in medicine.[11-16] The researchers seem perplexed that some patients prefer combination treatment with T_3 along with T_4; after all, the body is supposed to convert T_4 to the active hormone T_3. It appears, however, that variations in the gene that controls this conversion might explain why patients don't always react as doctors expect.[17]

There are many patients who prefer treatment with the very old-fashioned drug desiccated thyroid gland, available as Armour Thyroid, Naturethroid, Qualitest, Thyroid by Erfa (from Canada), or Westhroid. Although there have been occasional shortages, some form of thyroid extract is often available from compounding pharmacies who make products especially to match the patient's prescription. This preference can create conflict between patients and their physicians, as many physicians are reluctant to prescribe this type of thyroid hormone treatment. Like any thyroid treatment, desiccated thyroid requires periodic testing to ensure that the dose is appropriate. It seems, though, that a refusal even to consider this treatment, especially for a patient who has found it helpful in the past, might be a screwup.

Doctors are not the only ones who can make mistakes in thyroid treatment. Some patients have unrealistic expectations for what the treatment should do for them. Although it is very difficult for a hypothyroid person to lose weight, it is not reasonable to imagine that simply taking thyroid hormone of whatever description will make pounds melt away like magic. Weight loss still takes effort, and maintaining a good energy level still requires attention to proper nutrition, exercise, and adequate rest. What thyroid treatment does is remove the lead overshoes.

Another error patients sometimes make is to swallow their levothyroxine pills in the morning with their breakfast coffee and all their vitamin and mineral supplements.[18] Iron and calcium, as well as fiber-rich foods and espresso coffee, interfere with levothyroxine absorption,[19] and grapefruit juice reduces levothyroxine availability.[20] Levothyroxine is absorbed best on an empty stomach, at least half an hour before eating or drinking anything besides water. (If you get up early enough to give yourself time for this, well and good. If not, you could consider taking it at bedtime, at least two hours after eating anything. A Dutch study showed better results when levothyroxine was taken at bedtime,[21] although consistency is actually the most important issue when it comes to taking your thyroid pills.)

Another screwup, though one that is sometimes beyond the patient's control, is to shift from one generic form of levothyroxine to another. Although these drugs are all supposed to be acceptable, they aren't necessarily interchangeable and may not all behave in an identical fashion for every person. If you find one manufacturer's product works well for you, stick with it if at all possible. That way, you may save yourself and the doctor the trouble of additional testing and adjusting the dose.

Speaking of adjusting the dose, some people feel better if the dose of levothyroxine is adjusted seasonally, so that they take less in the summer and a bit more in the winter.[22] This is probably not well known by most doctors treating hypothyroidism, since the studies seem to focus on rather extreme circumstances like the Arctic Circle and Antarctica. Close doctor-patient cooperation makes it fairly easy to adjust dosage seasonally, however, without much danger.

One last mistake that patients would do well to avoid is to decide to just stop taking their thyroid medicine. Lots of people hate taking pills—who can blame them? Sometimes folks decide they'd rather treat their hypothyroidism with a natural product like seaweed. This is a big mistake. While it may, in rare circumstances, be possible to discontinue thyroid hormones, this should be done only in partnership with the physician and under close supervision. There are no herbs or dietary supplements that can take the place of thyroid hormone. To learn more about how some alternative therapies, including some supplements, can be added to the regimen, we recommend Mary Shomon's book *Living Well with Hypothyroidism.*

MIGRAINE HEADACHE

Migraines are miserable. In addition to pain that may be incapacitating, light and noise are very upsetting, and so are smells. Sufferers often feel the need to retreat to a dark, quiet room. Nausea is frequently part of the migraine picture, and the migraineur may be too nauseated to swallow a pill. He, or more commonly she, may be unable to concentrate well enough to drive or work or even hold a coherent conversation. The migraine can be traced to a biochemical disorder in the brain that seems to start with inflammation.

According to Joel Saper, MD, FACP, FAAN, founder and director of the Michigan Head-Pain and Neurological Institute, up to 4 percent of Americans experience this type of head pain commonly. Some people get migraine headaches every day. The sad thing is that daily migraines are sometimes the result of a screwup, either by the doctor or by the patient.

As Dr. Saper has pointed out,[1] doctors treating patients in pain are eager to relieve it. When they prescribe medications for pain, they may not impress upon the patient that a triptan migraine medicine such as sumatriptan (Imitrex), rizatriptan (Maxalt), or zolmitriptan (Zomig) should not be used more than two, or in extraordinary circumstances, three times a week. That guideline holds for other sorts of pain relievers as well, including over-the-counter pills for migraine. When a person starts to use any of these drugs more frequently, there is a danger of a rebound effect. This can lead to daily headaches and make the pain more resistant to treatment. It is not unusual for a patient to rely too heavily on over-the-counter analgesics and use them too frequently. Ultimately, this ends up causing the very headaches she was seeking to relieve.[2] It may be important to use other sorts of approaches to prevent or treat migraines so that one particular type of medication is not overused.[3]

Interactions are a potential problem with medications used to treat migraines. Doctors may prescribe a preventive medicine to be used daily. Beta blockers such as atenolol (Tenormin), propranolol (Inderal), or timolol (Blocadren) are sometimes used for this purpose, but propranolol may raise blood levels of rizatriptan (Maxalt) and exacerbate side effects such as dizziness, fatigue, nausea, and chest pain. Although antidepressants such as fluoxetine (Prozac) or sertraline (Zoloft) may be prescribed, their use is not well supported by research.[4] Such medications may, however, interact with triptan-type medicines, triggering an episode of serotonin syndrome (see page 96). Other medications that may be used preventively, such as topiramate (Topamax) or botulinum toxin (Botox) injection,[5] seem less susceptible to such interaction dangers.

One other mistake that is sometimes made in the treatment of migraine headaches is prescribing migraine-specific drugs such as the triptans or ergotamine-related medicines for middle-aged or older people with heart disease.[6] These drugs can trigger blood vessel contraction or spasm that can be extremely dangerous in such vulnerable patients, leading to a heart attack.[7]

Patients who soldier on without bringing their debilitating headaches to a doctor's attention may be playing with fire. Occasionally, a severe headache is a harbinger of more serious medical problems (such as a stroke or brain tumor) that need to be addressed. Unless there is a full diagnostic workup, that won't be discovered. As a result, being too stoic and not mentioning the migraines to the doctor could be a serious patient screwup.

OSTEOPOROSIS

For years, women have been warned about the hazards of fragile bones from osteoporosis as they grow older. For the most part, men have been given a pass. That might be the very first screwup when it comes to osteoporosis—women are being screened and treated too early (and possibly too much), and men at risk are not being recognized. But bone loss can affect men as well as women, particularly when men are treated with androgen blockers for prostate cancer.

Now, we don't mean to downplay the importance of osteoporosis. According to the National Institutes of Health, this deterioration of the structure of bone results in 1.5 million fractures a year.[1] Most of these are among elderly people, and about 300,000 of them are hip fractures. When an older person (whether female or male) breaks a hip, the recovery period is likely to be long and difficult. Complications are common, and 25 to 30 percent of hip fracture victims die within a few years.[2-3] So osteoporosis definitely merits attention, but jumping on the bisphosphonate bandwagon prematurely is a screwup.

This bandwagon is one that the pharmaceutical companies have encouraged. Starting in 1995, when Fosamax was introduced, there have been marketing campaigns aimed at getting women to take bisphosphonate drugs like risedronate (Actonel), ibandronate (Boniva), alendronate (Fosamax), and zoledronic acid (Reclast) starting in their fifties and sixties.[4] If women start taking these drugs soon after menopause, they might continue on for thirty or forty years. The TV ads and public service announcements have been successful: nearly $3.5 billion was spent on bisphosphonate drugs in 2008.[5]

The problem is that there are potential downsides to the bisphosphonates, especially when they are taken for many years. These drugs work by slowing bone breakdown. Bones may be hard, but they are living tissue, constantly being remodeled by cells that break old bone down (osteoclasts) and others that build new bone back (osteoblasts). The bisphosphonates put the brakes on the osteoclasts, so bone density is improved. But are the bones really stronger? Certain complications, especially jaw bone death (osteonecrosis of the jaw) and atypical fractures of the femur, or thigh bone, suggest that bisphosphonate-treated bone may be denser but not healthier. Both these complications are considered rare, but they should give providers and patients pause.

Fragile Femur

"In December 2007, my wife had been having pain in her right hip. Then on the twentieth, she walked into the bank lobby, turned right, and the right femur broke a couple of inches below her hip replacement prosthesis. Three surgeries were required to repair it. She had been taking Fosamax for ten to twelve years. Now her doctor has her taking Reclast."

We've suggested that these drugs are being marketed so that many more people (mostly women) are taking them than is truly warranted. This results from treating a number. When women undergo a bone density test, the test result is a number telling how much less dense the bones are than those of a thirty-year-old woman. Frequently, this number reveals that a postmenopausal woman has some bone loss, or osteopenia. The idea of preventing frank osteoporosis, or brittle bones, appeals to a lot of people, and that is probably why so many have been convinced to start taking medication to treat the osteopenia.

While we are definitely in favor of prevention, we'd suggest that the most beneficial preventive efforts when osteopenia is diagnosed might be both less expensive and less likely to cause side effects. A regular exercise regimen of walking, running, dancing, tennis, or anything that requires feet to hit the ground is one of the better ways to build bone strength. The earlier one starts exercising, the better, though people in their seventies and eighties can still get a great deal of benefit from an exercise program.

Maintaining a reasonable level of vitamin D, perhaps by doing some of that exercise outside in the summertime, is another preventive measure that seems to have little downside and may benefit bone strength in the long run.[6-7] There has been a great deal of emphasis on calcium, and it is important to get enough calcium. But how much calcium is enough is a topic that is currently under quite a bit of debate by medical researchers. A meta-analysis of fifteen clinical studies caused quite a stir when the researchers announced that "calcium supplements (without co-administered vitamin D) are associated with an increased risk of myocardial infarction [heart attack]."[8] The final word on calcium's benefits and risks is not in.

It is a mistake to concentrate solely on the bisphosphonates as though they were the only medicines available to treat osteoporosis. They may be the most heavily marketed, but there are other medications that are approved for treating osteoporosis. Be sure to discuss the pros and cons and long-term record of all of them with the prescribing physician. Ask about how long a drug can be used. Teriparitide (Forteo), for example, builds bone but it causes bone cancer in laboratory animals, so it should not be used for any longer than two years altogether. There is some evidence that four or five years of a bisphosphonate might be as good as ten, but there is much that is still unknown.[9] Older drugs such as calcitonin (Calcimar, Fortical, Miacalcin) or raloxifene (Evista) and newer ones such as denosumab (Prolia)[10] might also be relevant for certain patients, but people need to become well informed about possible risks and benefits for all these drugs, perhaps especially the newer agents, since there has been less time to discover potential problems.

One other screwup when it comes to osteoporosis is the long-term use of certain medications for other problems that can lead to bone loss and greater fracture risk. Sometimes the drugs are unavoidable, but doctors and patients should be alert to the potential for osteoporosis when patients must take medicines such as prednisone or other cortisone-like drugs for long periods of time.[11] A variety of other drugs can also increase the risk for fracture, including essential medications like anticonvulsants, antiandrogens for men being treated for prostate cancer, and aromatase inhibitors (anastrozole [Arimidex]; exemestane [Aromasin]; letrozole [Femara]) for women who have been treated for breast cancer. Anyone on a medication for an extended period of time should make sure to discuss it with the prescriber and learn what tactics should be undertaken to minimize the damage.

PROSTATE PROBLEMS

By the time they reach their later years, many men will find they need to get up several times a night to urinate. They may find that the stream is weak or slow and that it is difficult to completely empty the bladder. Along with this, many men experience a need to urinate immediately and may have to hurry to the bathroom.

While it might be logical to assume that these symptoms are connected to the kidneys, bladder, or other parts of the urinary tract, in fact they are most commonly due to an enlarged prostate gland. This male gland surrounds the urethra and produces some of the fluid that carries sperm during ejaculation. Years of exposure to a testosterone metabolite, dihydrotestosterone, make the prostate larger. This normal increase in size may reduce the amount of room for the urethra to pass through, resulting in the symptoms of benign prostatic hyperplasia (BPH).

One big mistake patients sometimes make is not to have the prostate checked when these symptoms become bothersome. Especially if they have suddenly worsened, or if there is blood in the semen or in the urine, symptoms typical of BPH might also be signaling prostate cancer. With troublesome symptoms, it definitely makes sense to see the doctor and find out what is causing them.

Benign Prostatic Hyperplasia (BPH)

If the symptoms are due to nothing more than the usual growth of the prostate gland with age (BPH), that's good news. But it doesn't mean it will be easy to figure out what to do to alleviate the problem. There are a lot of possible treatments, and the choice may be driven partly by personal preference or cost considerations. Most of the approaches seem to be roughly equivalent in effectiveness.

In years past, the man with severe urinary symptoms due to BPH would have been urged to go in for surgery. The usual surgical approach, transurethral resection of the prostate (TURP), usually reduced urinary symptoms, but it could result in complications. After the operation, some men suffered with incontinence or erectile dysfunction, a high price to pay for resolution of BPH symptoms.

That's probably why surgery is no longer the first-line approach for BPH.[1] Instead, most men are offered a prescription for a drug to alleviate symptoms, such as doxazosin (Cardura) or tamsulosin (Flomax), or a medication that slows or stops prostate enlargement, such as finasteride (Proscar) or dutasteride (Avodart). Sometimes men may take a combination of drugs, one from each of these categories.[2-4]

Although the studies suggest that the combinations may be more effective at relieving symptoms, there is the additional cost of two drugs as well as the increased risk of side effects that a man runs by taking two drugs instead of one. Drugs like tamsulosin (Flomax) or terazosin (Hytrin) can cause dizziness, weakness, nasal congestion, diminished libido, or a prolonged painful erection (this requires medical attention). In addition, men who may need cataract surgery in the future should be aware that such drugs can make the surgery more difficult because of a complication called intraoperative floppy iris syndrome.[5]

Finasteride and dutasteride can also cause sexual difficulties. One advantage of these drugs is that they appear to reduce the risk of a prostate cancer diagnosis if they are taken for a long period of time.[6-7] Men on either drug were about 25 percent less likely than those on a placebo to be diagnosed with prostate cancer, but there is one note of caution: both trials found that a somewhat higher proportion of the men diagnosed with prostate cancer had a more advanced tumor. It is unlikely that these drugs are causing prostate cancers to become more aggressive, but most experts admit there's not yet enough evidence to rule that possibility out completely.[8]

Some men might prefer nondrug approaches to treating their urinary symptoms. Certain herbs have been promoted for this purpose, but they have not been studied as well as the medications. Still, reviews of the research suggest that saw palmetto extract[9] and extract of an African plant called *Pygeum africanum*[10] may be useful for improving symptoms. Since herbal products are not regulated in the United States and may vary from one manufacturer to another, men who want to try them should look for evaluations of the products they are considering. One possible source is www.consumerlab.com.

Prostate Cancer

The wisdom of screening for prostate cancer in the absence of symptoms is still a matter of hot debate. Screening is usually done with a blood test for prostate-specific antigen (PSA). Using this marker can be tricky, however. Although PSA is specific to the prostate, it is not specific to prostate cancer. As a result, a single measurement does not tell very much. It is more helpful to see whether PSA levels are increasing and, if so, how rapidly. A man at high risk of prostate cancer due to a family history, for example, would be well advised to keep track of PSA levels at regular intervals. But someone with no particular risk factors might decide to leave well enough alone.

Why? That seems like a rather heretical statement, and of course it does not apply to someone who has new symptoms or a sudden increase in their severity. But an abnormal level of PSA doesn't necessarily mean prostate cancer. It could simply mean a big prostate. To check it out further, the doctor will do a biopsy. This procedure is a necessary step in the diagnosis of prostate cancer, but it is not completely without risk. And of course, if prostate cancer is discovered, the patient will have many decisions to make about treatment, beginning with the question of whether to treat it at all. Increasingly, doctors are considering the possibility of active surveillance (nicknamed "watch-and-wait") for prostate cancers that do not appear to be aggressive.[11] Analysis has shown that for some sixty-five-year-old men, this approach would result in a significant quality-of-life advantage without greatly increasing the risk of dying from prostate cancer.[12]

This approach might be especially appropriate for an older man. A friend of ours in his eighties with no particular symptoms saw a new-to-him (and probably inexperienced) internist, who ordered the PSA along with a range of other routine tests. When it came back high, she panicked and had a biopsy done on him within a few days. This resulted in a serious infection. The antibiotic that was prescribed induced a severe reaction. Our friend recovered, thank goodness, but it took him many months. Because the biopsy was positive for cancer, he was then treated with drugs that can cause hot flashes, digestive distress, and exhaustion. The natural history of prostate cancer suggests that a man in his mid-eighties is very likely to have cancer in his prostate gland, but unlikely to die from it soon. We'll never know if our friend suffered unnecessarily, but we suspect that might be the case. In our opinion, screening a healthy man over eighty for prostate cancer might be a screwup, and rushing him into surgery for the cancer he probably has could be another one.

On the other hand, urologist Mark McClure, MD, warns that one mistake patients may make is not taking a diagnosis of prostate cancer seriously enough. What does he mean? Basically, he is describing a man who just wants the doctor to tell him what treatment to use and then to rush through it. There is so much uncertainty about prostate cancer that there is no single "best" therapy; each man needs to become adequately informed about the pros and cons of the various treatments so that he can determine which one would be most appropriate in his particular case. The corresponding error on the physician's part is to assume that the patient is already well informed about the nature of prostate cancer and the range of treatment options available. That is often not the case, and both doctors and patients should build in time for the patient to do his homework and get up to speed. A delay of a few weeks while a man studies his options is hardly ever going to make a difference in the outcome of treatment for prostate cancer. This is not a good time to hurry.

It is really important to recognize that there are pros and cons for each possible way of treating prostate cancer. The very proliferation of treatments suggests that no one stands out from the others as the very best in all cases. Do keep in mind that doctors tend to prefer the type of treatment that they themselves provide, and be sure to seek out unbiased information about the potential benefits and risks. Many treatments for prostate cancer can have a negative impact on sexual function, for example. If this is important to you, make sure to ask about it and don't accept a brush-off.

If all this research is too overwhelming to do by yourself, enlist help. Some men may get a lot of assistance from their partners in asking questions and digging out resources. Others will need to look to friends, family members, or support groups. The one thing that is essential is to make sure you understand all your options so you can choose one you can live with. It may take time to read articles and interview several doctors, but it is time well spent.

TICK-BORNE DISEASES

When we talk about ticks, a lot of people think of Lyme disease. It is certainly true that Lyme disease is spread through a tick bite, but there are also a number of other possible infections that ticks can transmit. For the most part, doctors know how to treat these infections, which range from quite serious, in the case of Rocky Mountain spotted fever (RMSF),[1] to relatively mild, as in the case of southern tick-associated rash (STAR). The real opportunity for a screwup is in failing to diagnose the disease.

One problem is that the tick bite itself may have gone undetected. The second is that for some tick-borne diseases, such as RMSF or anaplasmosis, the initial infection starts with very nonspecific symptoms, rather flulike but not very distinctive.[2] Anaplasmosis, ehrlichiosis, and bartonellosis[3-5] are all better known as animal infections, but all can infect humans as well. Without a high index of suspicion, the doctor may not think of a tick-borne infection until the illness has become considerably more advanced. RMSF, for example, can be recognized in later stages by a distinctive rash, but not everyone develops a rash. Since RMSF can be a life-threatening infection, early diagnosis and treatment is especially important. (Despite the name, by the way, Rocky Mountain spotted fever is far more common in the southeastern states than in the Rockies.)

RMSF, anaplasmosis, and ehrlichiosis are all diseases that make you sick, and then you get better (unless, in the case of untreated RMSF, you die). According to Edward Breitschwerdt, DVM, one of the coun-try's leading experts on tick-borne and flea-borne infections, there's no evidence that any of the organisms that cause these diseases persist in the body and cause chronic problems. That is not true of *Borrelia burgdorferi*, the microbe that causes Lyme disease. This organism can cause chronic symptoms, both in animals and in humans. It may be even more difficult to think of a Lyme disease diagnosis if the patient does not live in an area where Lyme disease is common. (It is named Lyme disease after Old Lyme, a town in Connecticut where it was first identified. This disease is very common throughout New England and the Northeast into the upper Midwest, though it is now spreading into other parts of the country.) A person might visit New York or Vermont, return home to the Southeast, where Lyme is quite rare, and weeks later come down with a bull's-eye rash known as erythema migrans. If the doctor doesn't pick up on that, or if the patient does not develop the typical rash, months later the patient could have sore joints, overall aches, and fatigue and not know why.

The acute phase of Lyme disease usually responds well to antibiotics. If Lyme disease is not treated promptly and becomes chronic, however, its treatment is quite controversial. Because there is no good agreement, patients may become desperate and seek out a range of unusual thera-pies. Needless to say, this provides the opportunity for mistakes or mis-treatment. Scientists are actively pursuing a better understanding of the *Borrelia* bug and its behavior, and we can all hope that there will soon be a well-recognized way to cure chronic Lyme disease.

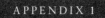

TOP 10 LIST OF POTENTIALLY PROBLEMATIC PILLS

We hesitate to create a list of problem drugs. The reason is that virtually *all* medications can cause side effects for *some* people. In many cases, such adverse drug effects can be life threatening. Does that mean these are bad drugs that should never be used? Of course not. Take chemotherapy, for example. Many chemo meds are highly toxic, with a long list of very serious side effects. But cancer is a life-threatening disease, and sometimes it takes a risky medicine to treat or cure a complicated condition. Most people are willing to take the chance of being treated with powerful drugs if they truly understand both the actual risks and the benefits of the drug they are being asked to take, especially if they are well informed about symptoms to watch for and actions to take if these symptoms occur. And that's the reason for this list. These are medications that require careful and close collaboration between patient, prescriber, and pharmacist.

The other serious flaw in creating a "problem" pill list is that it may give a false impression that drugs not on the list are somehow safe. That is absolutely *not* the case. There are thousands of very dangerous medicines on pharmacy shelves that can cause serious harm for some people, up to and including death. That said, we think that there are certain drugs that deserve more caution than others: even though they may play a very valuable, even life-saving role, they require extra vigilance. Another factor in our equation has to do with public perception. Some of the medications on our list are widely advertised and are taken by so many people that they may be taken for granted. When prescribers and patients let down their guard, it increases the possibility for screwups.

Our intent is not to scare anyone into stopping any of these pharmaceuticals. In fact, no one should *ever* stop taking any medication without the knowledge and approval of the prescriber. On the other hand, anyone who is taking such medications will need careful supervision and monitoring. We could easily have included fifty or more medications in this list, so please understand that this list is merely our opinion based on our years of researching and writing about drug safety. Were you to gather a hundred experts in pharmaceutical risk and ask them to put together their top-ten list of potentially problem drugs, you would likely get a lot of different opinions. We hope you, dear reader, will use this list thoughtfully to improve communication with both your prescriber and your pharmacist to help avoid medication misadventures.

1. **Anticoagulants.** Anticoagulants, drugs that are prescribed to reduce the likelihood of a blood clot, save lives. They prevent heart attacks, strokes, and other medical mischief. But medications such as warfarin (Coumadin) and clopidogrel (Plavix) can pose problems. In a 2010 study from the Inspector General of the Department of Health and Human Services, we learned that as many as 180,000 senior citizens die each year because of care they receive in hospitals.[1] Among the drugs that caused death in these Medicare recipients were blood thinners. The problem is usually excessive bleeding. Whenever an anticoagulant is prescribed, there is often a tightrope that has to be walked between blood clots on one hand and hemorrhage on the other. Add the very real possibility of drug interactions, and you have a recipe for risk. Anyone taking anticoagulants must be proactive to prevent problems.

2. **Digoxin (Digitek, Lanoxin, Lanoxicaps).** This heart medicine, which is derived from the plant digitalis, is one of the oldest and most interesting drugs in the pharmacy. It was used in its botanical form, foxglove, as far back as ancient Rome to treat heart failure. William Withering, MD, the father of digitalis medicine, brought the plant into mainstream medicine starting in 1785. The drug derived from the plant is still going strong after all this time. Over 10 million digoxin prescriptions were dispensed last year. And we have no doubt that this medicine still plays an important role in treating congestive heart failure and certain heart rhythm irregularities. The problem is that digoxin can be a

very tricky drug: the "margin of safety" between a safe dose and a toxic dose is very narrow. Symptoms of digitalis toxicity include loss of appetite, diarrhea, stomach pain, nausea, vomiting, visual disturbances (green or yellow tint and a halo around lights), weakness, apathy, depression, drowsiness, confusion, palpitations, rash, headaches, or hallucinations. Digoxin can interact dangerously with dozens of other drugs, so anyone taking digoxin must be monitored very carefully.

3. **Anti-inflammatory drugs (NSAIDs).** Americans are in a lot of pain. Surveys by the polling organization Roper and the National Consumers League estimate that over 20 million of us swallow a nonsteroidal anti-inflammatory drug (NSAID) like ibuprofen or naproxen every day. Hardly anyone heeds the warning to take over-the-counter pain relievers for no more than ten days without medical supervision. Only about one person in five reads the directions on the pain reliever label, and fewer than one in three bothers to check dosing instructions.[2] As a result, people get into all sorts of mischief with nonprescription NSAIDs. They also get into trouble with prescription pain relievers such as celecoxib (Celebrex); diclofenac (Cataflam, Voltaren); ibuprofen (Motrin); indomethacin (Indocin); ketorolac (Toradol); meloxicam (Mobic); naproxen (Naprosyn); oxaprozin (Daypro); and piroxicam (Feldene). Digestive upset (heartburn, stomach pain, nausea, constipation, diarrhea) is a common complaint. Bleeding ulcers, another complication, can be a life-threatening side effect. Over a decade ago, it was estimated that NSAIDs are responsible for 100,000 hospitalizations each year and 16,000 deaths.[3] That was before we learned that such drugs could also cause heart attacks and strokes. (Naproxen may be an exception to that complication.) Other adverse drug effects of NSAIDs include elevations in blood pressure, heart rhythm irregularities, fluid retention, dizziness, tinnitus, visual problems, headache, depression, skin rash, kidney, and liver damage. These drugs can also interact with dozens of other medications. NSAIDs must *not* be taken for granted, whether they are an over-the-counter brand like Advil or prescription-strength diclofenac.

4.   **Acetaminophen (APAP, or Tylenol).** Most Americans would be shocked to see acetaminophen on a problem pill list. It is perceived as one of the safest drugs in the pharmacy. That's in part because the manufacturer, McNeil, has presented the drug as super safe. During the 1980s, the company ran commercials emphasizing the phrase "trust Tylenol." Twenty years later, most patients don't think twice about Tylenol or house-brand acetaminophen. And yet accidental overdose is not uncommon. APAP (acetyl-para-aminophenol), the active compound in acetaminophen, is found in many different products, from cough and cold remedies to nighttime sleep aids. Many powerful prescription pain relievers such as Percocet and Vicodin contain acetaminophen.

Over 40,000 Americans end up in emergency rooms because of APAP overdoses. Food and Drug Administration (FDA) commissioner Margaret Hamburg, MD, offered the following remarks about acetaminophen on March 12, 2010: "This is an important medication that reduces the pain of millions of patients every day . . . but overdose is also the leading cause of acute liver failure and is responsible for hundreds of deaths each year. Shockingly, about half of people who overdosed did not intend to—they just took too much inadvertently. And this problem has gotten worse over the last decade."[4] Researchers have also discovered that just like NSAIDs, acetaminophen can raise blood pressure.[5-6] We suspect that is something few patients or physicians realize. There also appears to be an interaction between acetaminophen and warfarin that may increase the risk for dangerous or even fatal bleeding.[7-8] Bottom line: do not assume acetaminophen does not have side effects or take it for granted!

5.   **Narcotic analgesics (fentanyl; hydrocodone/APAP: Lorcet, Vicodin, Norco; oxycodone: Oxycontin; oxycodone/APAP: Percocet, Tylox).** Americans take an astonishing amount of narcotics. Known as opiates or opioids, such pain medicines are the most widely prescribed drugs in the United States. According to our calculations, almost 190 million prescriptions are filled each year for medications containing fentanyl, hydrocodone, methadone, and oxycodone. That does not in-

clude what is dispensed in hospitals and nursing homes. Please don't get us wrong. People in severe pain deserve adequate analgesia and should not fear opioid narcotics. Undertreatment of pain after surgery is a huge problem in many hospitals.[9] Cancer patients should never have to beg for pain relief.

That said, these drugs carry risks. For one thing, the most popular pills are a combination of either hydrocodone with acetaminophen, or oxycodone with acetaminophen. That means someone who needs a lot of medicine will be getting a big dose of acetaminophen (see discussion of APAP and liver damage on page 248). And there is also the potential for dependence. These drugs have been abused far too often. Getting the dose of narcotics right can be very tricky. Too much opioid can cause oversedation and "respiratory failure." In other words, you stop breathing. Narcotics are one of the most frequently implicated drugs in adverse reactions in hospitals.[10] Anyone taking such medicines or receiving opioids by injection needs to have an advocate double-checking the dose on a regular basis.

6. Corticosteroids (cortisone, dexamethasone, prednisolone, prednisone, methylprednisolone, etc.). When cortisone was first prescribed in 1949 to treat rheumatoid arthritis, it was called a wonder drug. Patients loved corticosteroids because they relieved pain and allowed people to function almost normally. During the 1950s, doctors felt like heroes when they prescribed drugs like prednisone because they worked like magic to ease many hard-to-treat conditions such as osteoarthritis, allergy, asthma, and atopic dermatitis. These drugs work by dampening inflammation and suppressing the immune system.

It took decades to learn about the dark side of corticosteroids. Long-term, high-dose use can cause cataracts, glaucoma, elevated blood pressure, potassium loss, blood clots, stomach ulcers, osteoporosis, diabetes, fluid retention, increased susceptibility to infections, high blood pressure, irregular heart rhythms, headache, menstrual disturbances, moon face, muscle weakness and wasting, bone deterioration, spontaneous fractures, insomnia, irritability, fatigue, and "steroid psychosis." Despite such complications, over 40 million prescriptions for corticosteroids were dispensed in retail pharmacies last year. In some cases, these drugs are lifesavers. When Joe developed sudden deafness in one ear, prednisone helped restore his hearing. We fear, however, that some physicians and patients have forgotten the lessons of the 1950s and are not giving such drugs the respect they deserve. Corticosteroids are still responsible for a great many adverse drug events each year.[11]

7. **Anti-arrhythmics for controlling irregular heart rates (amiodarone: Cordarone, Pacerone; dronedarone: Multaq).** There is no doubt that an irregular heart rhythm can be very scary and in some cases life threatening. Untreated atrial fibrillation, for example, can lead to blood clots that can cause a stroke. Selecting the best treatment for any given patient requires a knowledgeable cardiologist and great communication.

The history of antiarrhythmics has some serious speed bumps. In the mid-1980s, two drugs, encainide (Enkaid) and flecainide (Tambocor), were approved for treating heart rhythm disturbances. They were hailed as a major advance, and within a few years, 200,000 heart patients were taking either Enkaid or Tambocor. That success came to a screeching halt in 1989, however, when it was learned that people taking these medicines were dying faster than those on a placebo. The Cardiac Arrhythmia Suppression Trial (CAST) was halted prematurely because the results were so alarming.[12] Ever since this study, we have been very cautious when it comes to antiarrhythmic drugs.

Amiodarone carries a long list of possible side effects, including dizziness, serious visual problems, loss of appetite, nausea, fatigue, neuropathy, coordination problems, lung inflammation, liver toxicity, kidney failure, hypothyroidism, and heart failure. In some people, the arrhythmias actually worsen. Amiodarone can also interact with dozens of drugs in a dangerous way. A new drug, dronedarone, cannot be taken by patients with serious heart failure as it may make heart problems much worse. It, too, can interact with many medications and requires extreme vigilance to prevent serious complications.

8. **Atypical Antipsychotics (aripiprazole [Abilify]; olanzapine [Zy-prexa]; quetiapine [Seroquel]; risperidone [Risperdal]; ziprasidone [Geodon]).** The mentally ill have been tortured for centuries. People with schizophrenia have had holes drilled in their heads to let evil spirits escape. They have been starved, flogged, jailed, chained, and burned at the stake. In more "enlightened" times, they were put in straitjackets, wrapped in cold wet sheets, and locked in padded cells. Starting in 1946, patients were lobotomized, a procedure in which the frontal lobe of the brain was surgically destroyed with a tool like an ice pick.

Antipsychotic medications were a real advance over the barbaric treatments of prior decades. Drugs like chlorpromazine (Thorazine), haloperidol (Haldol), and thioridazine (Mellaril) were supposed to revolutionize the treatment of schizophrenia. Although they helped a bit with hallucinations, the side effects were nasty: uncontrollable muscle twitches or tics that were often irreversible, even after the drugs were stopped. Other side effects included blurred vision, nasal congestion, sexual problems, constipation, dry mouth, heart palpitations, dizziness, urinary retention, sedation, seizures, and a profound restlessness that made some people feel as if they wanted to jump out of their skin.

Enter a new generation of "atypical" antipsychotic medications in the 1990s. Drugs like Abilify, Risperdal, Seroquel, and Zyprexa were supposed to be much better than the nasty old head drugs from the 1950s and '60s. The hope was that not only would these medications be more effective, they would also be much safer. And they caught on like crazy, not just for schizophrenia but also for treating Alzheimer's and dementia, bipolar disorder, autism, obsessive-compulsive disorder, ADHD (attention deficit/hyperactivity disorder), insomnia and, major depression.

Despite the enthusiasm, though, a major study in the *New England Journal of Medicine* revealed that the newer, pricier atypical antipsychotics were no more effective for treating schizophrenia or less likely to cause troublesome side effects than an older antipsychotic.[13] Another study revealed an "increased risk of sudden cardiac death" associated with the atypicals.[14] An unexpected complication of these new-generation antipsychotics is substantial weight gain, which can lead to diabetes. Some other potential problems include drowsiness, dry mouth, headache, insomnia, dizziness, heartburn, tremor, elevated lipid levels, constipation, irregular heart rhythms, strokes, uncontrollable muscle movements, and blood disorders. Older people with dementia may be especially vulnerable to complications, including death.[15] For this reason, the FDA has required a black-box warning (a black-bordered warning on the package insert) that atypical antipsychotics are not approved for dementia-related psychosis. These drugs must be prescribed with great caution and monitored very carefully.

9. **Antidepressants (bupropion [Wellbutrin]; citalopram [Celexa]; desvenlafaxine [Pristiq]; duloxetine [Cymbalta]; escitalopram [Lexapro]; fluoxetine [Prozac, Serafem]; fluvoxamine [Luvox]; paroxetine [Paxil]; sertraline [Zoloft]; venlafaxine [Effexor]).** Depression is a terrible thing. It robs you of your zest for life. And with so many people feeling hopeless and helpless, it is no wonder that these drugs are prescribed in huge quantities. At the time of this writing, antidepressants were the fourth most prescribed class of drugs in America, with over 160 million prescriptions dispensed at a cost of roughly $10 billion.[16] With such an investment, you would expect these medications to be highly effective.

The most impressive study of antidepressant effectiveness was paid for by your tax dollars through the National Institutes of Health. The STAR*D trial (Sequenced Treatment Alternatives to Relieve Depression) examined actual recovery (remission) from depression. The results were remarkably disappointing. Despite exceptionally good care, only one in four patients actually achieved remission. With normal care, the numbers would have been far worse. Various meta-analyses of antidepressant drug trials have shown little, if any, benefit compared with a placebo.[17-20] See page 215 for more details about the controversy over antidepressant drug effectiveness.

Even though there are serious questions about the benefits of modern drugs for typical depression, we probably would not have included them on our list if they did not have problematic side effects. After years of controversy, the FDA required manufacturers of antidepressants to include a black-box warning about an increased risk of suicidal thoughts and actions in children, adolescents, and young adults. Other possible adverse drug events include nausea, loss of appetite, diarrhea, dry mouth, dizziness, fatigue, insomnia, tremor, anxiety, mania, low blood sugar, rash, visual disturbances, lowered libido, sexual dysfunction, seizures, low sodium levels, and a risk of bleeding. (Sexual dysfunction is not linked to bupropion.) When many of these antidepressants are stopped suddenly, there can be a kind of withdrawal reaction or "discontinuation syndrome" characterized by dizziness, nausea, sweating, chills, loss of appetite, or sensations like an electrical shock. Antidepressants can also interact with dozens of other drugs. Unless a person experiences meaningful benefit from such medications, these potential problems deserve respect.

10.   **Quinolone-type antibiotics (ciprofloxacin [Cipro, Proquin XR];** **levofloxacin [Levaquin]; moxifloxacin [Avelox]; norfloxacin [No-** **roxin]; ofloxacin [Floxin]).** Americans think of antibiotics as silver bullets. Given how penicillin changed medicine, that's not all that surprising. Most of us are so in awe of antibiotics that we rarely think of them as having side effects. A little stomach upset or temporary diarrhea is all we worry about. But some antibiotics can pose unexpected problems. The quinolone class of antibiotics can precipitate unusual problems for some people. One that may not be mentioned enough is tendinitis and tendon rupture. It was first recognized as a potential adverse effect in the early 1990s, but a black-box warning (FDA's highest-level caution) was not required until 2008. People over sixty and those taking corticosteroids are especially vulnerable, but even younger, healthy people can experience this devastating complication.

Another unexpected side effect of such antibiotics is central nervous system toxicity. This neurotoxic effect can manifest itself as anxiety, agitation, confusion, dizziness, depression, insomnia, headache, seizures, hallucinations, and even psychosis. How long the tendon damage or neurotoxic effects may linger remains controversial. Other worrisome complications may include skin rash, irregular heart rhythms, and long-lasting diarrhea brought on by a superinfection caused by *Clostridium difficile (C. diff.)*. This can also be a serious side effect of another antibiotic called clindamycin (Cleocin). Bottom line: these antibiotics have benefits, but they also have some serious side effects.

Other Problem Pills

As we stated in the introduction to this appendix, there are many other medications that can pose significant problems. Not included in our top 10 list are anticholinergic drugs prescribed to older people (see page 164), but they certainly belong here. Chemotherapy is always challenging. We also worry quite a lot about the stop-smoking pill varenicline (Chantix). One might think that any drug that helps people quit cigarettes is worth the problems, but we have received so many horror stories about Chantix on our website that we think this drug must be used very cautiously. And although many cardiologists think statins are so wonderful they should be in the water supply, we have heard too many reports of severe muscle and memory problems to think these are perfectly benign drugs. We are also concerned about the overprescribing of proton pump inhibitors (PPIs like Aciphex, Nexium, Prevacid, Prilosec, Protonix) for routine heartburn and bisphosphonates (Actonel, Boniva, Fosamax, Reclast) for something called osteopenia (low bone mineral density). Finally, management of diabetes is tricky. Whether the treatment is insulin or oral medicine, the goal must be to keep blood sugar in the sweet spot—neither too high nor too low.

All the drugs listed here and so many more require very careful supervision. Never take *any* medicine for granted.

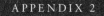

TOP 10 TIPS AND QUESTIONS LISTS

We have devoted most of this book to screwups by physicians, pharmacists, and other health care providers. We have alerted you to the many dangers that await us all when we seek a diagnosis or treatment. Just pointing out the problems without offering solutions would be pointless as well as depressing. In each chapter, we have tried to provide the tools that will empower you to prevent problems and improve outcomes.

There are many caring and compassionate health professionals who want very much to work with engaged patients to facilitate healing. Even providers who are caught up in the old paradigm can often be nudged in the right direction if you know what questions to ask and how to encourage their empathy and openness. We have collected all our tips and questions in this appendix for easy reference. In many cases, you will want to go back to the text for more context. There are some themes that repeat themselves. They include such ideas as to be assertive, take notes, make allies, have an advocate, ask for help, and be vigilant. We hope you find our top 10 tips and questions helpful as you interact with a dysfunctional health care system.

Top 10 Tips to Stopping Screwups in Hospitals (page 22)

1. Expect mistakes.
2. Drug-check.
3. Be assertive.
4. Say no!
5. Track transitions.
6. Call "Condition H" (Help).
7. Deal with discharge.
8. Cultivate communication.

9. Double-check everything.
10. Take a friend or family member.

Top 10 Screwups Doctors Make (page 27)

1. Not listening to patients
2. Misdiagnosing
3. Providing too little information
4. Not dealing with side effects
5. Undertreating or ignoring the evidence
6. Overtreating or being seduced by numbers
7. Overlooking drug interactions
8. Failing to revise the plan
9. Overlooking lab results
10. Not addressing lifestyle issues

Top 10 Diagnostic Screwups (page 44)

1. Pulmonary embolism (blood clot in lungs)
2. Drug reaction or overdose
3. Lung cancer
4. Colorectal cancer
5. Acute coronary syndrome (including heart attack)
6. Breast cancer
7. Strokes
8. Congestive heart failure
9. Fractures, various types
10. Abscesses

Top 10 Reasons Why Doctors Screw Up Diagnoses (page 46)

1. Overconfidence
2. Information overload
3. Going it alone
4. Tunnel vision
5. Time pressure
6. Missing test results
7. Ignoring drug side effects
8. Follow-up failure
9. Hurried hand-offs
10. Communication breakdown

Top 10 Questions to Ask to Reduce Diagnostic Disasters (page 69)

1. What are my primary concerns and symptoms?
2. How confident are you about this diagnosis?
3. What further tests might be helpful to improve your confidence?
4. Will the test(s) you are proposing change the treatment plan in any way?
5. Are there any findings or symptoms that don't fit your diagnosis or that contradict it?
6. What else could it be?
7. Can you facilitate a second opinion by providing me my medical records?
8. When should I expect to see my test results? Will you call with them, or will they come by mail or electronically?
9. What resources can you recommend for me to learn more about my diagnosis?
10. May I contact you by e-mail if my symptoms change or if I have an important question? If so, what is your e-mail address?

Top 10 Screwups Doctors Make When Prescribing (page 78)

1. Failing to disclose drug side effects
2. Creating obstacles to reporting symptoms
3. Ignoring drug-induced symptoms
4. Overriding medication alerts
5. Being oblivious to drug prices
6. Not knowing actual drug effectiveness
7. Relying on surrogate markers
8. Not checking for drug interactions
9. Not staying up to date on new research
10. Not reporting drug problems to the FDA

Top 10 Questions to Ask Your Doctor When You Get a Prescription (page 95)

1. Is there another way to treat my condition besides this drug?
2. What is the evidence that this drug will produce a meaningful outcome, not just change numbers on a test?
3. How likely am I to get a benefit from this medication?
4. What are the most common side effects?
5. What are the most serious side effects?
6. What symptoms require me to contact you immediately?
7. How can I get through to you promptly?
8. How long do I need to take this medication?
9. How should I take this drug—with food or without, morning or evening?
10. Are there any special instructions for stopping this medicine?

Top 11 Tips for Preventing Dangerous Drug Interactions (page 108)

1. Take a list of all your medicines to your appointment.
2. Find out how to take your medicine!
3. Check about whether any foods or beverages should be avoided.
4. Ask your doctor to check for interactions.
5. Ask your pharmacist to check for interactions.
6. Inquire about over-the-counter drugs.
7. Go to the Web to check on interactions yourself.
8. Don't take herbs or dietary supplements without checking for interactions.
9. Beware of drug-alcohol interactions.
10. Inquire about drug-disease interactions.
11. Check for prescription drug effects on laboratory test results.

Top 10 Screwups Pharmacists Make (page 111)

1. Not counseling patients
2. Dispensing the wrong drug
3. Dispensing the wrong dose
4. Ignoring interactions
5. Not standing up to doctors
6. Trusting all generic drugs
7. Relying on inadequate labels and leaflets
8. Not reporting errors
9. Switching drugs without patient approval
10. Not supervising techs carefully

Top 10 Tips for Taking Generic Drugs (page 139)

1. Make no assumptions.
2. Keep track of the manufacturer.
3. Keep records.
4. Ask for your lab results.
5. Monitor symptoms.
6. Listen to your body.
7. Challenge and rechallenge.
8. Be assertive.
9. Seek allies.
10. Report any problems to the Food and Drug Administration.

Top 10 Tips to Surviving Old Age (page 167)

1. Make sure your doctor *likes* older people.
2. Find a good geriatrician.
3. Ask about special dosing requirements.
4. Beware bad drugs (check the Beers List).
5. Avoid anticholinergic drugs if possible.
6. Minimize the number of drugs you take.
7. Seek nondrug treatment when practical.
8. Be assertive.
9. Have an advocate.
10. Stay active.

Top 10 Screwups Patients Make (page 168)

1. Not telling your story
2. Relying on memory
3. Not doing your homework
4. Skipping instructions

5. Not checking the prescription
6. Trusting all generic drugs
7. Overlooking lifestyle opportunities
8. Not seeking a second opinion
9. Not reading the fine print
10. Not asking for help

Questions to Ask Your Doctor Before Agreeing to Surgery (page 177)

1. What exactly will be done?
2. Why has it been recommended?
3. What are the alternatives?
4. What kind of anesthesia will be used?
5. What are the pros and cons of the procedure?
6. What are the pros and cons of the anesthesia?
7. What would happen if I opt out of the procedure?
8. What is the name of the doctor or surgeon who will be doing the procedure?
9. Who will be administering the anesthesia?
10. Will there be any other medical staff or learners present?
11. What will they be doing?
12. What are the pros and cons of any medication I will be given?
13. Are there any symptoms that are so serious they require immediate action?

Top 10 Tips to Promote Good Communication (page 188)

1. Find out when to arrive.
2. Be on time.
3. Ask for clarification of diagnoses and treatments.
4. Take notes.

5. Be clear about your previous treatment experience (know your body).

6. Keep records.

7. Target Web research carefully.

8. Follow up on test results.

9. Coordinate your other doctors' recommendations.

10. Do the homework on alternative approaches.

SAFE PATIENT CHECKLIST

✓ Take a prioritized list of your top health concerns/symptoms.

✓ Ask the doctor for a recap to make sure you have been heard.

✓ Take notes or record the conversation: you won't remember everything you have heard.

✓ Take a friend or family member to be your advocate and record keeper.

✓ Get a list of all your medications and supplements so that interactions can be prevented.

✓ Find out about the most common and serious side effects your medications may cause.

✓ Ask the doctor how confident he or she is about your diagnosis. Find out what else could cause your symptoms.

✓ When in doubt, seek a second opinion.

✓ Always ask your providers to wash their hands before they examine you.

✓ Get your medical records and test results.

✓ Keep track of your progress: maintain a diary of relevant measurements such as weight, blood pressure, and blood sugar readings.

✓ Be especially vigilant when moving from one health care setting to another. Mistakes and oversights are especially common during transitions.

✓ Ask how to get in touch with your providers. Get phone numbers or e-mail addresses, and learn when to report problems.

✓ Inquire about resources to learn more about your diagnosis or treatment.

Notes

SAFE PATIENT CHECKLIST

1. Classen, D. C., et al. " 'Global Trigger Tool' Shows That Adverse Events in Hospitals May Be Ten Times Greater Than Previously Measured." *Health Affairs* 2011; 30:581–589.

CHAPTER 1: INTRODUCTION

1. Centers for Disease Control and Prevention website. Accessed July 14, 2011. Mortality statistics for 2009, the latest available at the time of this writing.

2. Kohn, L. T., et al. *To Err Is Human: Building a Safer Health System.* Washington, DC: National Academies Press, 1999.

3. Leape, L. L., and Berwick, D. M. "Five Years After *To Err Is Human:* What Have We Learned?" *JAMA* 2005; 293:2384–2390.

4. HealthGrades Quality Study: "Patient Safety in American Hospitals," July 2004. www.healthgrades.com/media/english/paf/hg_patient_safety_study_final.pdf.

5. Hearst Corporation. *Dead by Mistake.* Aug. 9, 2009. www.chron.com/deadby mistake/.

6. Levinson, D. R. "Adverse Events in Hospitals: National Incidence Among Medicare Beneficiaries." Department of Health and Human Services, Office of Inspector General. Nov. 2010, OEI-06-09-00090.

7. *Dead by Mistake,* op. cit.

8. Grady, D. "Study Finds No Progress in Safety at Hospitals." *New York Times,* Nov. 24, 2010.

9. Nalder, E. "Detective Work Required to Uncover Errors." Hearst Newspapers, March 21, 2010. http://www.hearst.com/press-room/pr-20090809b.php.

10. Levinson, D. R. "Adverse Events in Hospitals: Case Study of Incidence Among Medicare Beneficiaries in Two Selected Counties," Department of Health and Human Services, Office of Inspector General, Dec. 2008. OEI-06-08-00220.

11. Landrigan, C. P., et al. "Temporal Trends in Rates of Patient Harm Resulting from Medical Care." *N. Engl. J. Med.* 2010; 363:2124–2134.

12. Ibid.

13. Goodman, J. C., et al. "The Social Cost of Adverse Medical Events, and What We Can Do About It." *Health Affairs* 2011; 30: 590–595.

14. Nalder, op. cit.

15. Milch, C. E., et al. "Voluntary Electronic Reporting of Medical Errors and

Adverse Events: An Analysis of 92,547 Reports from 26 Acute Care Hospitals." *J. Gen. Intern. Med.* 2006; 21:165–170.

16. Lopez, L., et al. "Disclosure of Hospital Adverse Events and Its Association with Patients' Ratings of the Quality of Care." *Arch. Intern. Med.* 2009; 169:1888–1894.

17. Classen, D. C., et al. " 'Global Trigger Tool' Shows That Adverse Events in Hospitals May Be Ten Times Greater Than Previously Measured." *Health Affairs* 2011; 30:581–589.

18. Bonello, R. S., Fletcher, C. E., et al. "An Intensive Care Unit Quality Improvement Collaborative in Nine Department of Veterans Affairs Hospitals: Reducing Ventilator-Associated Pneumonia and Catheter-Related Bloodstream Infection Rates." *Jt. Comm. J. Qual. Patient Saf.* 2008; 34:639–645.

19. *People's Pharmacy* radio show interview with Peter Pronovost, MD, PhD, March 24, 2010.

20. Hayward, R. A., et al. "Sins of Omission: Getting Too Little Medical Care May Be the Greatest Threat to Patient Safety." *J. Gen. Intern. Med.* 2005; 20:686–691.

21. Johnson, J. A., and Bootman, J. L. "Drug-Related Morbidity and Mortality and the Economic Impact of Pharmaceutical Care." *Am. J. Health-Syst. Pharm.* 1997; 54:554–558.

22. Lazarou, J., et al. "Incidence of Adverse Drug Reactions in Hospitalized Patients: A Meta-Analysis of Prospective Studies." *JAMA* 1998; 279:1200–1205.

23. Johnson, J. A., and Bootman, J. L. op. cit. *Am. J. Health-Syst. Pharm.* 1997; 54:554–558.

24. Bootman, J. L. "Drug-Related Morbidity and Mortality: An Economic and Clinical Perspective." *Managed Care* 2002; 11(2 Suppl.):12–15.

25. Kaiser Family Foundation State Health Facts.org website. http://www.statehealthfacts.org/comparemaptable.jsp?cat=8&ind=408. Accessed Jan. 18, 2011.

26. Bootman, J. L., et al. "The Health Care Cost of Drug-Related Morbidity and Mortality in Nursing Facilities." *Arch. Intern. Med.* 1997; 157:2089–2096.

27. Newman-Toker, D. E., and Pronovost, P. J. "Diagnostic Errors—The Next Frontier for Patient Safety." *JAMA* 2009; 301:1060–1062.

28. Shojania K. G., et al. "Changes in Rates of Autopsy-Detected Diagnostic Errors Over Time: A Systematic Review." *JAMA* 2003; 289:2849–2856.

29. Wachter, R. M. "Entering the Second Decade of the Patient Safety Movement: The Field Matures." *Arch. Intern. Med.* 2009; 169:1894–1896

30. Wachter, R. M. Personal communication (e-mail, Jan. 11, 2011): "A bit of a stretch to multiple deaths/year in the US (2.5 million) × 9% to come out with an estimate of mortality from diagnostic errors, but that would be one way of going about it."

31. Agency for Healthcare Research and Quality. "National Healthcare Quality Report 2009." AHRQ Publication No. 10–0003, March 2010.

32. "Nosocomial Infections: Challenges in Vaccine Development." New York Academy of Sciences online, Jan. 27, 2010. Presented by the Vaccine Science Discussion Group. www.nyas.org/events/detail.aspx?cid=e33d7d3e-4d89-4fb3-b54b-fc35e2b4c40e.

33. Richards, C. "Healthcare-Associated Infections: A Primer." Presented at "Toward the Elimination of Healthcare-Associated Infections," National Center for Preparedness, Detection, and Control of Infectious Diseases, Public Health Grand Rounds, Office of the Director, Oct. 15, 2009, Centers For Disease Control and Prevention. www.cdc.gov/about/grand-rounds/archives/2009/download/GR-101509.pdf.

34. Richards, op. cit. http://www.cdc.gov/about/grand-rounds/archives/2009/download/GR-101509.pdf; http://www.usatoday.com/news/health/2010-03-20-c-diff-bacteria_N.htm; Weise, E. "Lesser-known C-diff a Bigger Hospital Threat Than MRSA?" *USA Today*, March 22, 2010. http://www.todayshospitalist.com/index.php?b=articles_read&cnt=1021. Gesensway, D. "C.difficile, not MRSA, Is Now the Leading Pathogen in Some Hospitals." *Today's Hospitalist*, July 2010.

35. Berrington de Gonzalez, A., et al. "Projected Cancer Risks from Computed Tomographic Scans Performed in the United States in 2007." *Arch. Intern. Med.* 2009; 169:2071–2077.

36. Starfield, B. "Is US Health Really the Best in the World?" *JAMA* 2000; 284:483–485.

37. Leape, L. L. "Unnecessary Surgery." *Health Serv. Res.* 1989; 24:351–407.

38. Zhan, C., and Miller, M. R. "Excess Length of Stay, Charges, and Mortality Attributable to Medical Injuries During Hospitalization." *JAMA* 2003; 290:868–874.

39. Weingart, S. N., and Iezzoni, L. I. "Looking for Medical Injuries Where the Light Is Bright." *JAMA* 2003; 290:1917–1919.

40. Kim, E. S. H., and Bartholomew, J. R. "Venous Thromboembolism." http://www.clevelandclinicmeded.com/medicalpubs/diseasemanagement/cardiology/venous-thromboembolism. Accessed Jan. 15, 2011.

41. Beckman, M.G., et al. "Venous Thromboembolism: A Public Health Concern." *Am. J. Prev. Med.* 2010; 38(4S):S495-S501.

42. Heit, J. A., et al. "Estimated Annual Number of Incident and Recurrent, Non-Fatal and Fatal Venous Thromboembolism (VTE) Events in the U.S." *Blood* 2005; 106:267A.

43. Heit, J. A. "Venous Thromboembolism: Disease Burden, Outcomes and Risk Factors." *J. Thromb. Haemost.* 2005; 3:1611–1617.

44. Heit, J. A., et al. "Relative Impact of Risk Factors for Deep Vein Thrombosis and Pulmonary Embolism: A Population-Based Study." *Arch. Intern. Med.* 2002; 162:1245–1248.

45. Spyropoulos, A. C., and Lin, J. "Direct Medical Costs of Venous Thromboembolism and Subsequent Hospital Readmission Rates: An Administrative Claim Analysis from 30 Managed Care Organizations." *J. Manag. Care Pharm.* 2007; 13:475–486.

46. "Medication Error Reports," FDA update April 30, 2009. http://www.fda.gov/Drugs/DrugSafety/MedicationErrors/ucm080629.htm. Accessed April 29, 2010.

47. Weingart, S. N., et al. "Epidemiology of Medical Error." *BMJ* 2000; 320:774–777.

48. Ibid.

49. Gandhi, T. K., et al. "Adverse Drug Events in Ambulatory Care." *N. Engl. J. Med.* 2003; 348:1556–1564.

50. Centers for Disease Control and Prevention. "Estimates of Healthcare-Associated Infections." Cited in National Healthcare Quality Report 2009, US Department of Health and Human Services, Agency for Healthcare Research and Quality, AHRQ Publication No. 10-0003, March 2010. Issued on April 13, 2010.

51. Johnson, J. A., and Bootman, J. L. "Drug-Related Morbidity and Mortality and the Economic Impact of Pharmaceutical Care." *Am. J. Health-Syst. Pharm.* 1997; 54:554–558.

52. IOM Report Brief: *Preventing Medication Errors.* National Academies Press, July 2006.

53. Ibid.

54. Moyen, E., Camiré, E., and Stelfox, H. T. "Clinical Review: Medication Errors in Critical Care." *Critical Care* [BioMedCentral] 2008; 12:208. http://ccforum.com/content/12/2/208. Accessed April 13, 2011.

55. Weingart, S., et al. "Patient-Reported Medication Symptoms in Primary Care." *Arch. Intern. Med.* 2005; 165:234–240.

56. Ibid.

57. Classen, D. C., Jaser, L., and Budnitz, D. S. "Adverse Drug Events among Hospitalized Medicare Patients: Epidemiology and National Estimates from a New Approach to Surveillance." *Jt. Comm. J. Qual. Patient Saf.* 2010; 36(1):10–11.

58. Levinson, 2010, op. cit.

59. Encinosa, W. E., and Hellinger, F. J. "The Impact of Medical Errors on 90-Day Costs and Outcomes: An Examination of Surgical Patients." *Health Services Research* 2008; 43(6):2067–2085.

60. Barie, P. S. "Infection Control Practices in Ambulatory Surgical Centers." *JAMA* 2010; 303:2295–2297.

61. Schaefer, M. K., et al. "Infection Control Assessment of Ambulatory Surgical Centers." *JAMA* 2010; 303:2273–2279.

62. Leape, L. L. "Scope of Problem and History of Patient Safety." *Obstet. Gynceol. Clin. N. Am.* 2008; 35: 1–10.

63. Muder, R. R., et al. "Implementation of an Industrial Systems-Engineering Approach to Reduce the Incidence of Methicillin-Resistant Staphylococcus Aureus Infection." *Infect. Control Hosp. Epidemiol.* 2008; 29:702–708.

64. Crowley, C. F., and Nalder, E. "Within Healthcare Hides Massive, Avoidable Death Toll." Hearst Newspapers, *Dead by Mistake*, Aug. 10, 2009.

65. Pelt, J. L., and Faldmo, L. P. "Physician Error and Disclosure." *Clin. Obstet. Gynecol.* 2008; 51:700–708.

66. Kachalia, A., et al. "Liability Claims and Costs Before and After Implementation of a Medical Error Disclosure Program." *Ann. Intern. Med.* 2010; 153:213–221.

67. Loren, D. J., et al. "Medical Error Disclosure Among Pediatricians: Choosing Carefully What We Might Say to Parents." *Arch. Pediatr. Adolesc. Med.* 2008; 162:922–927.

68. Gallagher, T. H., et al. "Disclosing Harmful Medical Errors to Patients." *N. Engl. J. Med.* 2007; 356:2713–2719.

69. Gibson, R., Singh, J. P. *Wall of Silence: The Untold Story of the Medical Mistakes That Kill and Injure Millions of Americans.* Washington, DC: Lifeline Press, 2003.

70. Bates, D. W. "Drugs and Adverse Drug Reactions: How Worried Should We Be?" *JAMA* 1998; 279:1216–1217.

71. Wachter, R. M. "Patient Safety at Ten: Unmistakable Progress, Troubling Gaps." *Health Affairs* 2010; 29(1): 165–173.

72. Kilbridge, P. M., et al. "Automated Surveillance for Adverse Drug Events at a Community Hospital and an Academic Medical Center." *J. Am. Med. Inform. Assoc.* 2006; 13:372–377.

73. Wachter, R. M., and Pronovost, P. J. "Balancing 'No Blame' with Accountability in Patient Safety." *N. Engl. J. Med.* 2009; 361:1401–1406.

74. Ibid.

75. Ibid.

76. Ibid.

77. DesRoches, C. M., et al. "Physicians' Perceptions, Preparedness for Reporting, and Experiences Related to Impaired and Incompetent Colleagues." *JAMA* 2010; 304:187–193.

78. Garbutt, J., et al. "Reporting and Disclosing Medical Errors: Pediatricians' Attitudes and Behaviors." *Arch. Pediatr. Adolesc. Med.* 2007; 161:179–185.

79. Loren, op. cit.

80. Ibid.

81. Lamb, R. M., et al. "Hospital Disclosure Practices: Results of a National Survey." *Health Affairs* 2003; 22:73–83.

82. Gallagher, op. cit.

83. Lopez, L., et al. "Disclosure of Hospital Adverse Events and Its Association with Patients' Ratings of the Quality of Care." *Arch. Intern. Med.* 2009; 169:1888–1894.

84. IOM Report Brief, op. cit.

85. Ibid.

86. Flynn, E. A., et al. "National Observational Study of Prescription Dispensing Accuracy and Safety in 50 Pharmacies." *J. Am. Pharm. Assoc.* 2003; 43:191–200.

87. Casalino, L. P., et al. "Frequency of Failure to Inform Patients of Clinically Significant Outpatient Test Results." *Arch. Intern. Med.* 2009; 169(12):1123–1129.

CHAPTER 2: TOP 10 SCREWUPS DOCTORS MAKE

1. Ashbury, F. D., Iverson, D. C., and Kralj, B. "Physician Communication Skills: Results of a Survey of General/Family Practitioners in Newfoundland." *Med. Educ. Online* 2001; 6: 1–13. http://www.med-ed-online.org/res00014.htm. Accessed April 25, 2011.

2. Rhoades, D. R., et al. "Speaking and Interruptions During Primary Care Office Visits." *Fam. Med.* 2001; 33:(7):528–532.

3. Rhodes, K. V., et al. "Resuscitating the Physician-Patient Relationship: Emergency Department Communication in an Academic Medical Center." *Ann. Emerg. Med.* 2004; 44:262–267.

4. Rosenberg, E. E., et al. "Lessons for Clinicians from Physician-Patient Communication Literature." *Arch. Fam. Med.* 1997; 6:279–283.

5. Groopman, J. *How Doctors Think.* Boston: Houghton Mifflin, 2007, p. 35.

6. Newman-Toker, D. E., and Pronovost, P. J. "Diagnostic Errors—The Next Frontier for Patient Safety." *JAMA* 2009; 301:1060–1062.

7. Ibid.

8. *People's Pharmacy* radio show interview with David Newman-Toker, MD, PhD, and Peter Pronovost, MD, PhD, Aug. 29, 2009.

9. Rosenberg, op cit.

10. Rhodes, op. cit.

11. Weingart, S. N., et al. "Patient-Reported Medication Symptoms in Primary Care." *Arch. Intern. Med.* 2005; 165:234–240.

12. Ibid.

13. CDC Chronic Disease Indicators: Heart Failure Fact Sheet, Jan. 2010. http://www.cdc.gov/dhdsp/data_statistics/fact_sheets/docs/fs_heart_failure.pdf

14. Pitt, B., et al. "Randomized Aldactone Evaluation Study Investigators: The Effect of Spironolactone on Morbidity and Mortality in Patients with Severe Heart Failure." *N. Engl. J. Med.* 1999; 341:709–717.

15. Armstrong, P. W. "Aldosterone Antagonists—Last Man Standing?" *N. Engl. J. Med.* 2011; 364:79–80.

16. Albert, N. M., et al. "Use of Aldosterone Antagonists in Heart Failure." *JAMA* 2009; 302:1658–1665.

17. Ward, T. F., et al. "Statins for the Primary Prevention of Cardiovascular Disease." Cochrane Reviews online, Jan. 19, 2011. http://www2.cochrane.org/reviews/en/ab004816.html. Accessed April 25, 2011.

18. Green, L. A. "Cholesterol-Lowering Therapy for Primary Prevention." *Arch. Intern. Med.* 2010; 170:1007–1008.

19. Action to Control Cardiovascular Risk in Diabetes Study Group. "Effects of Intensive Glucose Lowering in Type 2 Diabetes." *N. Engl. J. Med.* 2008; 358:2545–2559.

20. ACCORD Study Group. "Effects of Intensive Blood-Pressure Control in Type 2 Diabetes Mellitus." *N. Engl. J. Med.* 2010; 362:1575–1585.

21. ACCORD Study Group. "Effects of Combination Lipid Therapy in Type 2 Diabetes Mellitus." *N. Engl. J. Med.* 2010; 362:1563–1574.

22. Qata, D. M., et al. "Use of Prescription and Over-the-Counter Medications and Dietary Supplements Among Older Adults in the United States." *JAMA* 2008; 300:2867–2878.

23. Isaac, T., et al. "Overrides of Medication Alerts in Ambulatory Care." *Arch. Intern. Med.* 2009; 169:305–311.

24. Yu, K., et al. "Prescribers' Knowledge of and Sources of Information for Potential Drug-Drug Interactions: A Postal Survey of US Prescribers." *Drug Safety* 2008; 31:525–536.

25. Pronovost, Peter, and Vohr, Eric. *Safe Patients, Smart Hospitals: How One Doctor's Checklist Can Help Us Change Health Care from the Inside Out.* New York: Hudson Street Press, 2010, pp. 31–35.

26. Casalino, L. P., et al. "Frequency of Failure to Inform Patients of Clinically Significant Outpatient Test Results." *Arch. Intern. Med.* 2009; 169:1123–1129.

27. Kvaavik, E., et al. "Influence of Individual and Combined Health Behaviors on Total and Cause-Specific Mortality in Men and Women: The United Kingdom Health and Lifestyle Survey." *Arch. Intern. Med.* 2010; 170:711–718.

28. *People's Pharmacy* extended radio show interview with Eric Westman, MD, May 1, 2010.

CHAPTER 3: DIAGNOSTIC DISASTERS

1. Zwaan, L., et al. "Patient Record Review of the Incidence, Consequences and Causes of Diagnostic Adverse Events." *Arch. Int. Med.* 2010; 170:1015–1021.

2. Fasano, A., et al. "Prevalence of Celiac Disease in At-Risk and Not-At-Risk Groups in the United States: A Large Multicenter Study." *Arch. Intern. Med.* 2003; 163: 286–292.

3. Rubio-Tapia, A., et al. "Increased Prevalence and Mortality in Undiagnosed Celiac Disease." *Gastroenterology* 2009; 137:88–93.

4. Newman-Toker, D. E., and Pronovost, P. J. "Diagnostic Errors—The Next Frontier for Patient Safety." *JAMA* 2009; 301:1060–1062.

5. Kohn, L. T., et al. *To Err Is Human: Building a Safer Health System.* Washington, D.C.: National Academies Press, 1999.

6. Graber, M. "Diagnostic Errors in Medicine: A Case of Neglect." *Jt. Comm. J. Qual. Patient Saf.* 2005; 31:106–113.

7. Wachter, R. M. "Diagnostic Errors Don't Get Any Respect—And What Can Be Done About Them." *Health Affairs* 2010; 29:1605–1610.

8. *People's Pharmacy* radio show interview with Peter Pronovost, MD, PhD, March 24, 2010.

9. Schiff, G. D., et al. "Diagnostic Error in Medicine." *Arch. Intern. Med.* 2009; 169:1881–1887.

10. Leonhardt, D. "Why Doctors So Often Get It Wrong." *New York Times*, Feb. 22, 2006.

11. Lundberg, G. D. "Low-Tech Autopsies in the Era of High-Tech Medicine: Continued Value for Quality Assurance and Patient Safety." *JAMA* 1998; 280:1273–1274.

12. Nichols, L., et al. "Are Autopsies Obsolete?" *Am. J. Clin. Pathol.* 1998; 110:210–218.

13. Elstein, A. S. "Clinical Reasoning in Medicine." In: Higgs, J. J. M., ed. *Clinical Reasoning in the Health Professions.* Oxford, England: Butterworth-Heinemann Ltd., 1995.

14. Berner, E. S., and Graber, M. L. "Overconfidence as a Cause of Diagnostic Error in Medicine." *Am. J. Med.* 2008; 121:S2–S23.

15. Schiff, op cit.

16. Ibid.

17. Gandhi, T. K., et al. "Missed and Delayed Diagnoses in the Ambulatory Setting: A Study of Closed Malpractice Claims." *Ann. Intern. Med.* 2006; 145:488–496.

18. Kachalia, A., et al. "Missed and Delayed Diagnoses in the Emergency Department: A Study of Closed Malpractice Claims from 4 Liability Insurers." *Ann. Emerg. Med.* 2007; 49:196–205.

19. Philips, R. L., Jr., et al. "Learning from Malpractice Claims About Negligent, Adverse Events in Primary Care in the United States." *Qual. Saf. Health Care* 2004; 13:121–126.

CHAPTER 4: TOP 10 REASONS WHY DOCTORS SCREW UP DIAGNOSES

1. Haskell, Meg. "Bangor Doctor Touts New Diagnostic Technology." *Bangor Daily News,* Aug. 23, 2008.

2. Gawande, A. "The Velluvial Matrix." *New Yorker,* June 16, 2010.

3. Jacobs, Lee. "Interview with Lawrence Weed, MD—The Father of the Problem-Oriented Medical Record Looks Ahead." *Permanente Journal* 2009; 13:84–90.

4. Graber, M. "Diagnostic Errors in Medicine: A Case of Neglect." *Jt. Comm. J. Qual. Patient Saf.* 2005; 31:106–113.

5. Berner, E. S., and Graber, M. L. "Overconfidence as a Cause of Diagnostic Error in Medicine." *Am. J. Med.* 2008; 121:S2–S23.

6. Ibid.

7. Ibid.

8. Podbregar, M., et al. "Should We Confirm our Clinical Diagnostic Certainty by Autopsies?" *Intensive Care Med.* 2001; 27:1750–1755.

9. Friedman, C.P., et al. "Do Physicians Know When Their Diagnoses Are Correct?" *J. Gen. Intern. Med.* 2005; 20:334–339.

10. Potchen, E. J. "Measuring Observer Performance in Chest Radiology: Some Experiences." *J. Am. Coll. Radiol.* 2006; 3:423–432.

11. Graber, M., op. cit.

12. *People's Pharmacy* radio show interview with Peter Pronovost, MD, PhD, March 24, 2010.

13. Centor, R. M. "Expand the Pharyngitis Paradigm for Adolescents and Young Adults." *Ann. Intern. Med.* 2009; 151:812–815.

14. Sanders, Lisa. "The Strep Throat That Wasn't." *New York Times Magazine,* Sept. 14, 2008.

15. Sanders, Lisa. *Every Patient Tells a Story: Medical Mysteries and the Art of Diagnosis.* New York: Broadway Books, 2009, pp. 30–32.

16. Newman-Toker, D. E., and Pronovost, P. J. "Diagnostic Errors—The Next Frontier for Patient Safety." *JAMA* 2009; 301:1060–1062.

17. *People's Pharmacy* interview with Peter Pronovost, op. cit.

18. Bauer, B. A., et al. "Internal Medicine Resident Satisfaction with a Diagnostic Decision Support System (DXplain) Introduced on a Teaching Hospital Service." *Proc. AMIA Symp.* 2002; 31–35.

19. Rosenbloom, S. T., et al. "Effect of CPOE User Interface Design on User-Initiated Access to Educational and Patient Information During Clinical Care." *J. Am. Med. Inform. Assoc.* 2005; 12:458–473.

20. Berner, E. S., op. cit.

21. Teich, J. M., et al. "Effects of Computerized Physician Order Entry on Prescribing Practices." *Arch. Intern. Med.* 2000; 160:2741–2747.

22. Garg, A. X., et al. "Effects of Computerized Clinical Decision Support Systems on Practitioner Performance and Patient Outcomes: A Systematic Review." *JAMA* 2005; 293:1223–1238.

23. Maguire, P. "Is an Access Crisis on the Horizon in Mammography?" *ACP Observer* 2003; 23:1. http://www.acpinternist.org/archives/2003/10/mammo.htm. Accessed April 13, 2011.

24. Groopman, Jerome. *How Doctors Think.* Boston: Houghton Mifflin, 2007, p. 65.

25. Coulehan, op. cit.

26. Salgo, Peter. "The Doctor Will See You for Exactly Seven Minutes." *New York Times,* March 22, 2006.

27. Casalino, L. P., et al. "Frequency of Failure to Inform Patients of Clinically Significant Outpatient Test Results." *Arch. Intern. Med.* 2009; 169:1123–1129.

28. Ibid.

29. Harper, Matthew. "How Many People Take Cholesterol Drugs?" *Forbes,* Oct. 30, 2008.

30. Kausik, K. R., et al. "Statins and All-Cause Mortality in High-Risk Primary Prevention." *Arch. Intern. Med.* 2010; 170:1024–1031.

31. Golomb, B. A., et al. "Physician Response to Patient Reports of Adverse Drug Effects: Implications for Patient-Targeted Adverse Effect Surveillance." *Drug Safety* 2007; 30:669–675.

32. Golomb, B. A. "Implications of Statin Adverse Effects in the Elderly: Editorial." *Expert Opin. Drug Saf.* 2005; 4:389–397.

33. Phillips, P. S., et al. "Statin-Associated Myopathy with Normal Creatine Kinase Levels." *Ann. Intern. Med.* 2002; 137:581–585.

34. Joy, T. R., and Hegele, R. A. "Narrative Review: Statin-Related Myopathy." *Ann. Intern. Med.* 2009; 150:858–868.

35. Mohaupt, M. G., et al. "Association Between Statin-Associated Myopathy and Skeletal Muscle Damage." *CMAJ* 2009; 181:E11–E18.

36. Gaist, et al. "Statins and Risk of Polyneuropathy: A Case-Control Study." *Neurology* 2002; 58:1333–1337.

37. Muldoon, M. F., et al. "Randomized Trial of the Effects of Simvastatin on Cognitive Functioning in Hypercholesterolemic Adults." *Am. J. Med.* 2004; 117:823–829.

38. Langsjoen, P. H., et al. "Treatment of Statin Adverse Effects with Supplemental Coenzyme Q10 and Statin Drug Discontinuation." *Biofactors* 2005; 25:147–152.

39. Golomb, B. A., and Evans, M. A. "Statin Adverse Effects: A Review of the Literature and Evidence for a Mitochondrial Mechanism." *Am. J. Cardiovasc. Drugs* 2008; 8:373–418.

40. Hippisley-Cox, J., and Coupland, C. "Unintended Effects of Statins in Men and Women in England and Wales: Population Based Cohort Study Using the QResearch Database." *BMJ* 2010; 340:c2197.

41. Graber, M. op. cit.

42. Kachalia, A., et al. "Missed and Delayed Diagnoses in the Emergency Department: A Study of Closed Malpractice Claims from 4 Liability Insurers." *Ann. Emerg. Med.* 2007; 49:196–205.

43. Schiff, G. D., et al. "Diagnostic Error in Medicine: Analysis of 583 Physician-Reported Errors." *Arch. Intern. Med.* 2009; 169:1881–1887.

44. USP Patient Safety CAPSLink: Miscommunication Leads to Confusion and Errors. http://www.usp.org/pdf/EN/patientSafety/capsLink2003-12-01.pdf. Accessed July 14, 2010.

45. Gandhi, T. K., et al. "Missed and Delayed Diagnoses in the Ambulatory Setting: A Study of Closed Malpractice Claims." *Ann. Intern. Med.* 2006; 145:488–496.

CHAPTER 5: PREVENTING DIAGNOSTIC PROBLEMS

1. *People's Pharmacy* radio show interview, with Peter Pronovost, MD, PhD, March 24, 2010.

2. Coulehan, J. "On Humility." *Ann. Intern. Med.* 2010; 153:200–201.

3. Pronovost, P. J., et al. "Sustaining Reductions in Catheter Related Bloodstream Infections in Michigan Intensive Care Units: Observational Study." *BMJ* 2010; 340:c309.

4. http://participatorymedicine.org/a-declaration-of-participation/. Accessed July 30, 2010. Definition from the Society for Participatory Medicine.

5. Coulehan, J. op. cit.

6. *People's Pharmacy* radio show interview with David Newman-Toker, MD, PhD, and Peter Pronovost, MD, PhD, Aug. 29, 2009.

7. Berrintton de Gonzalez, A., et al. "Projected Cancer Risks from Computed Tomographic Scans Performed in the United States in 2007." *Arch. Intern. Med.* 2009; 169:2071–2077.

8. Hoffman, R. M., and Zeliadt, S. B. "The Cautionary Tale of PSA Testing." *Arch. Intern. Med.* 2010; 170:1262–1263.

9. Sanders, Lisa. *Every Patient Tells a Story: Medical Mysteries and the Art of Diagnosis.* New York: Broadway Books, 2009, pp. 30–32.

10. Casalino, L. P., et al. "Frequency of Failure to Inform Patients of Clinically Significant Outpatient Test Results." *Arch. Intern. Med.* 2009; 169:1123–1129.

11. Greenwald, R. ". . . And a Diagnostic Test Was Performed." *N. Engl. J. Med.* 2005; 353:2089–2090.

12. Gerstle R. S. "E-mail Communication Between Pediatricians and Their Patients." *Pediatrics* 2004; 114:317–321.

13. Rosen, P., and Kwoh, C. K. "Patient-Physician E-mail: An Opportunity to Transform Pediatric Health Care Delivery." *Pediatrics* 2007; 120:701–706.

14. Ibid.

15. Ibid.

16. Zhou, Y. Y., et al. "Improved Quality at Kaiser Permanente Through E-mail Between Physicians and Patients." *Health Affairs* 2010; 29:1370–1375.

CHAPTER 6: TOP TEN SCREWUPS DOCTORS MAKE WHEN PRESCRIBING

1. IMS Health. "IMS Health Reports U.S. Prescription Sales Grew 5.1 Percent in 2009, to $300.3 Billion." Press release. www.imshealth.com. April 1, 2010.

2. Leone, R., et al. "Drug-Related Deaths." *Drug Safety* 2008; 31:703–713.

3. Johnson, J. A., and Bootman, J. L. "Drug-Related Morbidity and Mortality: A Cost-of-Illness Model." *Arch. Intern. Med.* 1995; 155:1949–1956.

4. Johnson, J. A., and Bootman, J. L. "Drug-Related Morbidity and Mortality and the Economic Impact of Pharmaceutical Care." *Am. J. Health-Syst. Pharm.* 1997; 54:554–558.

5. Lazarou, J., et al. "Incidence of Adverse Drug Reactions in Hospitalized Patients: A Meta-Analysis of Prospective Studies." *JAMA* 1998; 279:1200–1205.

6. IOM Report Brief: *Preventing Medication Errors*, National Academies Press, July 2006.

7. Weingart, S., et al. "Patient-Reported Medication Symptoms in Primary Care." *Arch. Intern. Med.* 2005; 165:234–240.

8. Lasser, K. E., et al. "Adherence to Black Box Warnings for Prescription Medications in Outpatients." *Arch. Intern. Med.* 2006; 166:338–344.

9. Weingart, op. cit.

10. Ibid.

11. Gandhi, T. K., et al. "Drug Complications in Outpatients." *J. Gen. Intern. Med.* 2000; 15:149–154.

12. Editorial: "Inform the Patient." *JAMA* 1970; 211:654.

13. Weingart, op. cit.

14. Ibid.

15. Hohl, C. M., et al. "Emergency Physician Recognition of Adverse Drug-Related

Events in Elder Patients Presenting to an Emergency Department." *Acad. Emerg. Med.* 2005; 12:197–205.

16. Hohl, C. M., et al. "Do Emergency Physicians Attribute Drug-Related Emergency Department Visits to Medication-Related Problems? *Ann. Emerg. Med.* 2010; 55:493–502.

17. Young, S. "FDA Launches Program to Prevent Errors in Medication Use." CNN Health, Nov. 4, 2009. http://www.cnn.com/2009/HEALTH/11/04/medication.misuse.fda/index.html. Accessed April 13, 2011.

18. Nicholson, D., et al. "Medication Errors: Not Just a Few Bad Apples." *J. Clin. Outcomes Manag.* 2006; 12:114–115.

19. Isaac, T., et al. "Overrides of Medication Alerts in Ambulatory Care." *Arch. Intern. Med.* 2009; 169:305–311.

20. Associated Press, "Drug Errors Injure More Than 1.5 Million a Year." July 29, 2006.

21. Bourgeois, F. T., et al. "Pediatric Adverse Drug Events in the Outpatient Setting: An 11-Year National Analysis." *Pediatrics* 2009; 124:e744–3750.

22. Schneider, E. L., and Campese, V. M. "Adverse Drug Responses: An Increasing Threat to the Well-Being of Older Patients." *Arch. Intern. Med.* 2010; 170:1148–1149.

23. Weingart, S. N., et al. "Medication Errors Involving Oral Chemotherapy." *Cancer* 2010; 116:2455–2464.

24. Allan, G. M., et al. "Physician Awareness of Drug Cost: A Systematic Review." *PLoS Med.* 2007; 4:e283.

25. Ibid.

26. Connor, S. "Glaxo Chief: Our Drugs Do Not Work on Most Patients." *The Independent/UK*, Dec. 8, 2003.

27. Fournier, J. C. "Antidepressant Drug Effects and Depression Severity: A Patient-Level Meta-Analysis." *JAMA* 2010; 303:47–53.

28. Vedantam, S. "Against Depression, a Sugar Pill Is Hard to Beat." *Washington Post*, May 7, 2002.

29. Kirsch, I., et al. "Initial Severity and Antidepressant Benefits: A Meta-Analysis of Data Submitted to the Food and Drug Administration." *PLoS Medicine* 2008; 5:e45.

30. Rubinow, D. R. "Treatment Strategies After SSRI Failure—Good News and Bad News." *N. Engl. J. Med.* 2006; 354:1305–1307.

31. Courtney, C., et al. "Long-Term Donepezil Treatment in 565 Patients with Alzheimer's Disease (AD2000): Randomised Double-Blind Trial." *Lancet* 2004; 363:2105–2115.

32. Wiysonge, C. S., et al. "Beta-Blockers for Hypertension." *Cochrane Database Syst. Rev.* 2007; CD002003.

33. Zhou, C. N., et al. "Calcium Channel Blockers Versus Other Classes of Drugs for Hypertension." *Cochrane Database Syst. Rev.* 2010; CD003654.

34. Wright, J. M., and Musini, V. M. "First-Line Drugs for Hypertension." *Cochrane Database Syst. Rev.* 2009; CD001841.

35. Bradley, H. A., et al. "How Strong Is the Evidence for Use of Beta-Blockers as First-Line Therapy for Hypertension? Systematic Review and Meta-Analysis." *J. Hypertens.* 2006; 24:2131–2141.

36. Carlberg, B., et al. "Atenolol in Hypertension: Is It a Wise Choice?" *Lancet* 2004; 364:1684–1689.

37. Aronow, W. S. "Current Role of Beta-Blockers in the Treatment of Hypertension." *Expert Opin. Pharmacother.* 2010; 11:S1–S9.

38. Green, L. A. "Cholesterol-Lowering Therapy for Primary Prevention: Still Much We Don't know." *Arch. Intern. Med.* 2010; 170:1007–1008.

39. Ray, K. K., et al. "A Meta-Analysis of 11 Randomized Controlled Trials Involving 65220 Participants." *Arch. Intern. Med.* 2010; 170:1024–1031.

40. Nissen, S. E., and Wolski, K. "Effect of Rosiglitazone on the Risk of Myocardial Infarction and Death from Cardiovascular Causes." *N. Engl. J. Med.* 2007; 356:2457–2471.

41. Rosen, C. J. "Revisiting the Rosiglitazone Story—Lessons Learned." *N. Engl. J. Med.* 2010; 363:803–805.

42. Graham, D. J., et al. "Risk of Acute Myocardial Infarction, Stroke, Heart Failure, and Death in Elderly Medicare Patients Treated with Rosiglitazone or Pioglitazone." *JAMA* 2010; 304:411–418.

43. Whalen, J., and Mundy, A. "FDA Scientist Attacks Avandia Safety." *Wall Street Journal*, June 11, 2010.

44. Isaac, op. cit.

45. Antoniou, T., et al. "Trimethoprim-Sulfamethoxazole-Induced Hyperkalemia in Patients Receiving Inhibitors of the Renin-Angiotensin System: A Population-Based Study." *Arch. Intern. Med.* 2010; 170:1045–1049.

46. Figueiras, A., et al. "An Educational Intervention to Improve Physician Reporting of Adverse Drug Reactions." *JAMA* 2006; 296:1086–1093.

47. Hazell, L., and Shakir, S. A. W. "Under-Reporting of Adverse Drug Reactions: A Systematic Review." *Drug Safety* 2006; 29:385–396.

CHAPTER 7: DRUG INTERACTIONS CAN BE DEADLY

1. FDA Patient Safety News: Show #54, October, 2006. "Warning on Combining Triptans and SSRIs/SNRI." http://www.accessdata.fda.gov/psn/printer.cfm?id=463. Accessed Nov. 13, 2010.

2. U.S. Food and Drug Administration. "Selective Serotonin/Norepinephrine Reuptake Inhibitors (SNRIs)." http://www.fda.gov/Safety/MedWatch/SafetyInformation/SafetyAlertsforHumanMedicalProducts/ucm150748.htm. Accessed Nov. 13, 2010.

3. Surdin, Ashley. "Coroner Attributes Michael Jackson's Death to Sedative." *Washington Post*, Aug. 25, 2009. http://www.washingtonpost.com/wp-dyn/content/article/2009/08/24/AR2009082402193.html. Accessed Nov. 13, 2010.

4. Yee, J. L., et al. "Drug-Related Emergency Department Visits in an Elderly Veteran Population." *Ann. Pharmacother.* 2005; 39:1990–1995.

5. Juurlink, D. N., et al. "Drug-Drug Interactions Among Elderly Patients Hospitalized for Drug Toxicity." *JAMA* 2003; 289:1652–1658.

6. Jankel, C. A., and Fitterman, L. K. "Epidemiology of Drug-Drug Interactions as a Cause of Hospital Admissions." *Drug Safety* 1993; 9:51–59.

7. Ko, Y., et al. "Potential Determinants of Prescribers' Drug-Drug Interaction Knowledge." *Res. Social Adm. Pharm.* 2008; 4:355–366.

8. Ko, Y., et al. "Prescribers' Knowledge of and Sources of Information for Potential Drug-Drug Interactions." *Drug Safety* 2008; 31:525–536.

9. Glassman, P. A., et al. "Improving Recognition of Drug Interactions: Benefits and Barriers to Using Automated Drug Alerts." *Medical Care* 2002; 40:1161–1171.

10. Langdorf, M. I., et al. "Physician Versus Computer Knowledge of Potential Drug Interactions in the Emergency Department." *Acad. Emerg. Med.* 2000; 7:1321–1329.

11. Dormann, H., et al. "Lack of Awareness of Community-Acquired Adverse Drug Reactions upon Hospital Admission: Dimensions and Consequences of a Dilemma." *Drug Safety* 2003; 26:353–362.

12. Antoniou, T., et al. "Trimethoprim-Sulfamethoxazole-Induced Hyperkalemia in Patients Receiving Inhibitors of the Renin-Angiotensin System." *Arch. Intern. Med.* 2010; 170:1045–1049.

13. Langdorf, op. cit.

14. Ko, op. cit.

15. Langdorf, op. cit.

16. Teich, J. M., et al. "Effects of Computerized Physician Order Entry on Prescribing Practices." *Arch. Intern. Med.* 2000; 160:2741–2747.

17. Bates, D. W., et al. "Effect of Computerized Physician Order Entry and a Team Intervention on Prevention of Serious Medication Errors." *JAMA* 1998; 280:1311–1316.

18. Abookire, S. A., et al. "Improving Allergy Alerting in a Computerized Physician Order Entry System." *Proc. AMIA Symp.* 2000: 2–6.

19. Monane, M., et al. "Improving Prescribing Patterns for the Elderly Through On-line Drug Utilization Review Intervention: A System Linking the Physician, Pharmacist and Computer." *JAMA* 1998; 280:1249–1252.

20. Public Citizen Worst Pills, Best Pills website: http://www.worstpills.org/public/page.cfm?op_id=4. Accessed April 13, 2011.

21. Kuhlmann, J., and Muck, W. "Clinical-Pharmacological Strategies to Assess Drug Interaction Potential During Drug Development." *Drug Saf.* 2001; 24:715–725.

22. Hohl, C. M., et al. "Do Emergency Physicians Attribute Drug-Related Emergency Department Visits to Medication-Related Problems?" *Ann. Emerg. Med.* 2010; 55:493–502.

23. Grizzle, A. J., et al. "Reasons Provided by Prescribers When Overriding Drug-Drug Interaction Alerts." *Am. J. Manag. Care* 2007; 13:573–580.

24. Judge, J., et al. "Prescribers' Responses to Alerts During Medication Ordering in the Long Term Care Setting." *JAMIA* 2006; 13:385–390.

CHAPTER 8: TOP 10 SCREWUPS PHARMACISTS MAKE

1. Rajecki, Ron. "Drug Topics' 2010 Pharmacists Salary Survey." *Drug Topics*, April 7, 2010.

2. "Pharmacy Technicians and Aides." *Occupational Outlook Handbook, 2010–2011 Edition.* Bureau of Labor Statistics.

3. Ibid.

4. Cina, J. L., et al. "How Many Hospital Pharmacy Medication Dispensing Errors Go Undetected?" *Jt. Comm. J. Qual. Patient Saf.* 2006; 32:73–80.

5. Flynn, E. A., et al. "National Observational Study of Prescription Dispensing Accuracy and Safety in 50 Pharmacies." *J. Am. Pharm. Assoc.* 2003; 43:191–200.

6. Flynn, E. A., et al. "Dispensing Errors and Counseling Quality in 100 Pharmacies." *J. Am. Pharm. Assoc.* 2009; 49:171–180.

7. Allan, E. L., et al. "Dispensing Errors and Counseling in Community Practice." *Am. Pharm.* 1995; ns35:25–33.

8. Ibid.

9. Flynn, 2009, op cit.

10. Ibid.

11. McCoy, K. "Lawsuit: Walgreens Prescription Error Killed Man." *USA Today*, November 2, 2007.

12. Baynews9.com "After Wrongful Death, Family Sues Walgreen's, Wins." March 2, 2010.

13. Headden, S., et al. "Danger at the Drugstore: Too Many Pharmacists Fail to Protect Consumers Against Potentially Hazardous Interactions of Prescription Drugs." *U.S. News & World Report*, Aug. 18, 1996.

14. Flynn, E. A., 2009, op. cit., p. 177.

15. Svarstad, B. L., et al. "Expert and Consumer Evaluation of Patient Medication Leaflets in U.S. Pharmacies." *J. Am. Pharm. Assoc.* 2005; 45:443–451.

16. Cina, op. cit., p. 75.

17. Hughes, C. M., et al. "Use of Medication Technicians in US Nursing Homes: Part of the Problem or Part of the Solution?" *J. Am. Med. Dir. Assoc.* 2006; 7:294–304.

CHAPTER 9: GENERIC DRUG SCREWUPS

1. U.S. Food and Drug Administration. "Generic Drugs: Questions and Answers: What Are Generic Drugs?" http://www.fda.gov/Drugs/ResourcesForYou/Consumers/QuestionsAnswers/ucm100100.htm. Accessed November 11, 2010.

2. Graedon, Joe. *The People's Pharmacy.* New York: St. Martin's Press, 1976, pp. 293–304.

3. Schmid, J. Personal communication, Nov. 25, 2002.

4. Buhay, N. Personal communication, Sept. 13, 2002.

5. Statement of Joshua M. Sharfstein, MD, FDA principal deputy commissioner, before the Subcommittee on Health, Committee on Energy and Commerce, House of Representatives (Washington, DC, March. 10, 2010).

6. Hamburg, M. A. "FDA and the American Public: The Safety of Foods and Medical Products in the Global Age." Remarks of Margaret A. Hamburg, MD, commissioner of Food and Drugs at Center for Strategic and International Studies, Feb. 4, 2010.

7. GAO, *Food and Drug Administration: Improvements Needed in the Foreign Drug Inspection Program.* GAO/HEHS-98-21 (Washington, DC: March 17, 1998).

8. GAO. *Drug Safety: Better Data Management and More Inspections Are Needed to Strengthen FDA's Foreign Drug Inspection Program.* GAO-08-970 (Washington, DC: Sept. 22, 2008).

9. GAO. *Drug Safety: FDA Has Conducted More Foreign Inspections and Begun to Improve Its Information on Foreign Establishments, but More Progress Is Needed.* GAO-10-961 (Washington, DC: Sept. 30, 2010).

10. Ibid.

11. Eban, Katherine. "Bad Bargain." *SELF,* June 2009.

12. Mundy, Alicia, "China Never Investigated Tainted Heparin, Says Probe." *Wall Street Journal,* July 22, 2010.

13. Moore, T. J., et al. QuarterWatch: 2008 Quarter 3, released May 7, 2009. *Institute for Safe Medication Practices.* http://www.ismp.org/quarterwatch/2008Q3.pdf. Accessed Nov. 8, 2010.

14. Okie, S. "Multinational Medicines—Ensuring Drug Quality in an Era of Global Manufacturing." *N. Engl. J. Med.* 2009; 361:737–740.

15. Ibid.

16. Ibid.

17. ConsumerLab.com. "Wellbutrin vs. Generic Bupropion." Initial Posting, Oct. 10, 2007; last updated, Dec. 2, 2009. https://www.consumerlab.com/reviews/Wellbutrin _vs_Generic_Bupropion/Wellbutrin. Accessed Nov. 10, 2010.

18. Beck, Melinda. "Inexact Copies: How Generics Differ from Brand Name." *Wall Street Journal,* April 22, 2008.

19. U.S. Food and Drug Administration. "Review of Therapeutic Equivalence Generic Bupropion XL 300 mg and Wellbutrin XL 300." Updated Sept. 18, 2009. http://www.fda.gov/AboutFDA/CentersOffices/CDER/ucm153270.htm. Accessed November 10, 2010.

20. Ibid.

21. Beck, op. cit.

22. Krauskopf, L., and Berkrot, B. "Generics to Cut U.S. Drugs Bill by $70 Billion." Reuters, Nov. 8, 2010.

23. Edney, Anne. "FDA Says It May Tighten Standards for Generic Drugs." *Bloomberg,* Oct. 10, 2010.

24. Loftus, Peter. "Whistleblower's Long Journey: Glaxo Manager's Discovery of Plant Lapses in '02 Led to Her $96 Million Payout." *Wall Street Journal*, Oct. 28, 2010.

CHAPTER 10: THE SCREWING OF SENIOR CITIZENS

1. US Census Bureau (2009) National Age and Sex Characteristics. http://www .census.gov/popest/national/asrh. Accessed Oct. 26, 2010.

2. Gallagher, P., et al. "Inappropriate Prescribing in the Elderly." *J. Clin. Pharmacy Ther.* 2007; 32:113–121.

3. Liu, G. G., and Christensen, D. B. "The Continuing Challenge of Inappropriate Prescribing in the Elderly: An Update of the Evidence." *J. Am. Pharm. Assoc.* 2002; 42:847–857.

4. Schneider, E. L., and Campese, V. M. "Adverse Drug Response." *Arch. Intern. Med.* 2010; 170:1148–1149.

5. Kaufman, D. W., et al. "Recent Patterns of Medication Use in the Ambulatory Adult Population of the United States: The Slone Survey." *JAMA* 2002; 287:337–344.

6. Goldberg, R. M., et al. "Drug-Drug and Drug-Disease Interactions in the Emergency Department: Analysis of a High-Risk Population." *Am. J. Emerg. Med.* 1996; 14:447–450.

7. Ramaswamy, R., et al. "Potentially Inappropriate Prescribing in Elderly: Assessing Doctor Knowledge, Confidence and Barriers." *J. Eval. Clin. Prac.* E-pub ahead of print July 13, 2010. http://onlinelibrary.wiley.com/doi/10.1111/j.1365-2753.2010.01494.x/ abstract.

8. Levinson, Daniel R. *Adverse Events in Hospitals: National Incidence Among Medicare Beneficiaries.* Health and Human Services, Office of Inspector General, Nov. 2010. OEI-06-09-00090. http://oig.hhs.gov/oei/reports/oei-06-09-00090.pdf. Accessed Nov. 1, 2010.

9. Schneider, op. cit.

10. Gurwitz, J. H., et al. "Incidence and Preventability of Adverse Drug Events Among Older Persons in the Ambulatory Setting." *JAMA* 2003; 289:1107–1116.

11. Goulding, M. R. "Inappropriate Medication Prescribing for Elderly Ambulatory Care Patients." *Arch. Intern. Med.* 2004; 164:305–312.

12. Ramaswamy, op. cit.

13. Kusserow, R. P. *Medicare Drug Utilization Review*, Office of Inspector General, April 1989. OAI-01-88-00980.

14. American Academy of Pediatrics website: http://www.aap.org/workforce/. Accessed Oct. 13, 2010.

15. Warshaw, G. A., et al. "Which Patients Benefit the Most from a Geriatrician's Care? Consensus Among Directors of Geriatrics Academic Programs." *J. Am. Geriatr. Soc.* 2008; 56:1796–1801.

16. *Retooling for an Aging America: Building the Health Care Workforce.* Institute of Medicine. http://iom.edu/Reports/2008/Retooling-for-an-Aging-America-Building -the-Health-Care-Workforce.aspx. Released April 11, 2008.

17. Rowe, John W. Statement Before the Special Committee on Aging, U.S. Senate, April 16, 2008.

18. Ibid.

19. Gross, Jane. "Geriatrics Lags in Age of High-Tech Medicine." *New York Times,* Oct. 18, 2006.

20. Boult, C., et al. "The Urgency of Preparing Primary Care Physicians to Care for Older People with Chronic Illnesses." *Health Aff. (Millwood).* 2010; 29:811–818.

21. Avorn, Jerry. "Medication Use in Older Patients: Better Policy Could Encourage Better Practice." *JAMA* 2010; 304:1606–1607.

22. Croasdale, Myrle. "Baby Boomer Time Bomb: Too Many Aging Patients, Too Few Geriatricians." *American Medical News* (amednews.com), May 5, 2008. www.ama-assn.org/amednews/2008/05/05/prl10505.htm. Accessed Oct. 16, 2010.

23. Gross, op. cit.

24. Avorn, op. cit.

25. Avila-Beltran, R., et al. "Geriatric Medical Consultation Is Associated with Less Prescription of Potentially Inappropriate Medications." *J. Am. Geriatr. Soc.* 2008; 56:1778–1779.

26. Hjemdahl, P., et al. "SBU Should Investigate What Is an Evidence-Based and Cost-Effective Use of Statins." *Lakartidningen* 2009; 106:1992–1994.

27. Petersen, L. K., et al. "Lipid-Lowering Treatment to the End? A Review of Observational Studies and RCTs on Cholesterol and Mortality in 80+-Year Olds." *Age Ageing* 2010; 39:674–680.

28. Goldstein, M. R., et al. "Statin Therapy in the Elderly: Misconceptions." *J. Am. Geriatr. Sc.* 2008; 56:1365.

29. Petersen, op. cit.

30. Noda, H., et al. "Low-Density Lipoprotein Cholesterol Concentrations and Death Due to Intraparenchymal Hemorrhage: The Ibaraki Prefectural Health Study." *Circulation* 2009; 119:2136–2145.

31. Huang, X, et al. "Low LDL Cholesterol and Increased Risk of Parkinson's Disease: Prospective Results from Honolulu-Asia Aging Study." *Mov. Disord.* 2008; 23:1013–1018.

32. Jacobs, D., et al. "Report of the Conference on Low Blood Cholesterol: Mortality Associations." *Circulation* 1992; 86:1046–1060.

33. Alsheikh-Ali, A. A., et al. "Effect of the Magnitude of Lipid Lowering on Risk of Elevated Liver Enzymes, Rhabdomyloysis, and Cancer." *J. Am. Coll. Cardio.* 2007; 50:409–418.

34. Yashin, A. I., et al. "Dynamic Determinants of Longevity and Exceptional Health." *Curr. Gerontol. Geriatr. Res.* E-pub ahead of print Sept. 30, 2010. pii: 3811637. http://www.ncbi.nlm.nih.gov/pmc/articles/PMC2952789/?tool=pubmed.

35. Beers, M., et al. "Psychoactive Medications Use in Intermediate-Care Facility Residents." *JAMA* 1988; 260:3016–3020.

36. Beers, M. H., et al. "Explicit Criteria for Determining Inappropriate Medication Use in Nursing Home Residents." *Arch. Intern. Med.* 1991; 151:1825–1832.

37. Fick, D. M., et al. "Updating the Beers Criteria for Potentially Inappropriate Medication Use in Older Adults: Results of a US Consensus Panel of Experts." *Arch. Intern. Med.* 2003; 163:2716–2724.

38. Wilcox, S. M., et al. "Inappropriate Drug Prescribing for the Community-Dwelling Elderly." *JAMA* 1994; 272:292–296.

39. Lund, B. C., et al. "Inappropriate Prescribing Predicts Adverse Drug Events in Older Adults." *Ann. Pharmacother.* 2010; 44:957–963.

40. Ramaswamy, op. cit.

41. Fick, op. cit.

42. Zuckerman, J. D. "Hip Fracture." *N. Engl. J. Med.* 1996; 334:1519–1525.

43. "Hip Fractures Among Older Adults." Centers for Disease Control and Prevention online. http://www.cdc.gov/ncipc/factsheets/adulthipfx.htm. Accessed Oct. 30, 2010.

44. De Vries, O. J. "Multifactorial Intervention to Reduce Falls in Older People at High Risk of Recurrent Falls." *Arch. Intern. Med.* 2010; 170:1110–1117.

45. Woolcott, J. C., et al. "Meta-Analysis of the Impact of 9 Medication Classes on Falls in Elderly Persons." *Arch. Intern. Med.* 2009; 169:1952–1960.

46. Weinblatt, M. E. "Nonsteroidal Anti-Inflammatory Drug Toxicity: Increased Risk in the Elderly." *Scand. J. Rheumatol. Suppl.* 1991; 91:9–17.

47. Hegeman, J., et al. "NSAIDs and the Risk of Accidental Falls in the Elderly: A Systematic Review." *Drug Safety* 2009; 32:489–498.

48. Farley, J. F., and Blalock, S. J. "Trends and Determinants of Prescription Medication Use for Treatment of Osteoporosis." *Am. J. Health-Syst. Pharm.* 2009; 66:1191–1201.

49. Sellmeyer, D. E. "Atypical Fractures as a Potential Complication of Long-Term Bisphosphonate Therapy." *JAMA* 2010; 304:1480–1484.

50. Shane, E., et al. "Atypical Subtrochanteric and Diaphyseal Femoral Fractures: Report of a Task Force of the American Society for Bone and Mineral Research." *J. Bone Miner. Res.* 2010; 25:2267–2294.

51. Wilkinson, G. S., et al. "Atrial Fibrillation and Stroke Associated with Intravenous Bisphosphonate Therapy in Older Patients with Cancer." *J. Clin. Oncol.,* 2010; 28:4898–4905.

52. Ancelin, M. L., et al. "Non-Degenerative Mild Cognitive Impairment in Elderly People and Use of Anticholinergic Drugs: Longitudinal Cohort Study." *BMJ* 2006; 332:455–459.

53. Doraiswamy, Murali P., and Gwyther, Lisa P. *The Alzheimer's Action Plan: The Experts' Guide to the Best Diagnosis and Treatment for Memory Problems.* New York: St. Martin's Press, 2008.

54. Carriere, I., et al. "Drugs with Anticholinergic Properties, Cognitive Decline, and Dementia in an Elderly General Population." *Arch. Intern. Med.* 2009; 169:1317–1324.

55. Scheife, R., and Takeda, M. "Central Nervous System Safety of Anticholinergic

Drugs for the Treatment of Overactive Bladder in the Elderly." *Clin. Ther.* 2005; 27:144–153.

56. Rudolph, J. L., et al. "The Anticholinergic Risk Scale and Anticholinergic Adverse Effects in Older Persons." *Arch. Intern. Med.* 2008; 168:508–513.

57. Ancelin, op. cit.

58. Padala, K. P., et al. "Simvastatin-Induced Decline in Cognition." *Ann. Pharmacother.* 2006; 40:1880–1883.

59. Galatti, L., et al. "Short-Term Memory Loss Associated with Rosuvastatin." *Pharmacotherapy* 2006; 26:1190–1192.

60. Golomb, B. A., et al. "Physician Response to Patient Reports of Adverse Drug Effects: Implications for Patient-Targeted Adverse Effect Surveillance." *Drug Safety* 2007; 30:669–675.

61. Wagstaff, L. R., et al. "Statin-Associated Memory Loss: Analysis of 60 Case Reports and Review of the Literature." *Pharmacotherapy* 2003; 23:871–880.

62. Muldoon, M. F., et al. "Randomized Trial of the Effects of Simvastatin on Cognitive Functioning in Hypercholesterolemic Adults." *Am. J. Med.* 2004; 117:823–829.

63. Evans, M. A., and Golomb, B. A. "Statin-Associated Adverse Cognitive Effects: Survey Results from 171 Patients." *Pharmacotherapy* 2009; 29:800–811.

CHAPTER 11: TOP 10 SCREWUPS PATIENTS MAKE

1. Ashbury, F. D., Iverson, D. C., and Kralj, B. "Physician Communication Skills: Results of a Survey of General/Family Practitioners in Newfoundland." *Med. Educ. Online* 2001; 6:1–13. http://www.med-ed-online.org/res00014.htm. Accessed April 13, 2011.

2. Rhoades, D. R., et al. "Speaking and Interruptions During Primary Care Office Visits." *Fam. Med.* 2001; 33(7):528–532.

3. Rhodes, K. V., et al. "Resuscitating the Physician-Patient Relationship: Emergency Department Communication in an Academic Medical Center." *Ann. Emerg. Med.* 2004; 44:262–267.

4. Rosenberg, E. E., et al. "Lessons for Clinicians from Physician-Patient Communication Literature." *Arch. Fam. Med.* 1997; 6:279–283.

5. Heffernan, V. "A Prescription for Fear." *New York Times Magazine*, Feb. 6, 2011, pp. 14–16.

6. Flynn, E. A., et al. "National Observational Study of Prescription Dispensing Accuracy and Safety in 50 Pharmacies." *J. Am. Pharm. Assoc.* 2003; 43:191–200.

7. Katz, M. H. "Failing the Acid Test: Benefits of Proton Pump Inhibitors May Not Justify the Risks for Many Users." *Arch. Intern. Med.* 2010; 170:747–748.

8. Ibid.

9. *People's Pharmacy* radio show interview with Peter Pronovost, MD, PhD, March 24, 2010.

10. Groopman, J. *Second Opinions: Stories of Intuition and Choice in the Changing World of Medicine.* New York: Viking Press, 2000.

11. Landro, Laura. "Consent Forms That Patients Can Understand." *Wall Street Journal*, Feb. 6, 2008.

12. Yap, T. Y., et al. "A Physician-Directed Intervention: Teaching and Measuring Better Informed Consent." *Acad. Med.* 2009; 84:1036–1042.

13. Meier, B. "Surgeon vs. Knee Maker: Who's Rejecting Whom?" *New York Times*, June 20, 2010.

14. IOM Report Brief: *Preventing Medication Errors.* National Academies Press, July 2006.

CHAPTER 12: CLOSING THE COMMUNICATION CHASM

1. Beck, Melinda. "The Doctor Will See You Eventually." *Wall Street Journal*, Oct. 18, 2010.

2. Weingart, S. N., Gandhi, T. K., et al. "Patient-Reported Medication Symptoms in Primary Care." *Arch. Intern. Med.* 2005(2); 165:234–240.

3. Roter, D. L., et al. "Can E-Mail Messages Between Patients and Physicians be Patient-Centered?" *Health Commun.* 2008; 23:80–86.

4. Houston, T. K., et al. "Experience of Patients Who Were Early Adopters of Electronic Communication with Their Physicians: Satisfaction, Benefits, and Concerns." *Am. J. Manag. Care* 2004; 10:601–608.

5. Houston, T. K., et al. "Experience of Physicians Who Frequently Use E-Mail with Patients." *Health Commun.* 2003; 15:515–525.

6. Patt, M. R., et al. "Doctors Who Are Using E-Mail with Their Patients: A Qualitative Exploration." *J. Med. Internet. Res.* 2003; 5:e9.

7. Halbert, S. C., French, B., et al. "Tolerability of Red Yeast Rice (2,400 mg Twice Daily) Versus Pravastatin (20 mg Twice Daily) in Patients with Previous Statin Intolerance." *Am J Cardiol.* 2010; 105(2):198–204.

CHAPTER 13: TOP SCREWUPS IN COMMON CONDITIONS

1. Vaughn, B. T., et al. "Can We Close the Income and Wealth Gap Between Specialists and Primary Care Physicians?" *Health Affairs* 2010; 29:933–940.

2. Zoungas, S., et al. "Severe Hypoglycemia and Risks of Vascular Events and Death." *N. Engl. J. Med.* 2010; 363:1410–1418.

3. Hippisley-Cox, J., and Coupland, C. "Unintended Effects of Statins in Men and Women in England and Wales: Population Based Cohort Study Using the QResearch Database." *BMJ* 2010; 340: c2197.

Acne

1. Haider, A., and Shaw, J. C. "Treatment of Acne Vulgaris." *JAMA.* 2004; 292(6):726–735.

2. Eichenfield, L. F., Jarratt, M., et al. "Adapalene 0.1% Lotion in the Treatment of Acne Vulgaris: Results from Two Placebo-Controlled, Multicenter, Randomized Double-Blind, Clinical Studies." *J. Drugs Dermatol.* 2010; 9(6):639–646.

3. Sagransky, M., Yentzer, B. A., and Feldman, S. R. "Benzoyl Peroxide: A Review of its Current Use in the Treatment of Acne Vulgaris." *Expert Opin. Pharmacother.* 2009; 10(15):2555–2562.

4. Ebede, T. L., Arch, E. L., and Berson, D. "Hormonal Treatment of Acne in Women." *J. Clin. Aesthet. Dermatol.* 2009; 2:16–22.

5. Cook, D., Krassas, G., and Huang, T. "Acne: Best Practice Management." *Aust. Fam. Physician* 2010; 39:656–660.

6. Ibid.

7. Patel, M., et al. "The Development of Antimicrobial Resistance due to the Antibiotic Treatment of Acne Vulgaris: A Review." *J. Drugs Dermatol.* 2010; 9(6):655–664.

8. Kinney, M. A., Yentzer, B. A., et al. "Trends in the Treatment of Acne Vulgaris: Are Measures Being Taken to Avoid Antimicrobial Resistance?" *J. Drugs Dermatol.* 2010; 9(5):519–524.

9. Gerding, D. N. "*Clostridium difficile* 30 Years On: What Has, or Has Not, Changed and Why?" *Int. J. Antimicrob. Agents.* 2009; 33 Suppl 1:S2–S8.

10. Fulton, James E., Jr., Plewig, Gerd, and Kligman, Albert M. "Effect of Chocolate on Acne Vulgaris." *JAMA* 1969; 210(11):2071–2074.

11. Wolf, R., Matz, H., and Orion, E. "Acne and Diet." *Clin. Dermatol.* 2004; 22 (5):387–393.

12. Rasmussen, J. E., and Smith, S. B. "Patient Concepts and Misconceptions About Acne." *Arch. Dermatol.* 1983; 119(7):570–572.

13. Cordain, L., Lindeberg, S., et al. "Acne Vulgaris: A Disease of Western Civilization." *Arch. Dermatol.* 2002; 138:1584–1590.

14. Jung, J. Y., Yoon, M. Y., et al. "The Influence of Dietary Patterns on Acne Vulgaris in Koreans." *Eur. J. Dermatol.* 2010; 20:768–772.

15. Melnik, B. C., and Schmitz, G. "Role of Insulin, Insulin-Like Growth Factor-1, Hyperglycaemic Food and Milk Consumption in the Pathogenesis of Acne Vulgaris." *Exp. Dermatol.* 2009; 18(10):833–841.

16. Berra, B., and Rizo, A. M. "Glycemic Index, Glycemic Load: New Evidence for a Link with Acne." *J. Am. Coll. Nutr.* 2009; 28 Suppl:450S-454S.

17. Melnik, B. C. "The Role of Transcription Factor FoxO1 in the Pathogenesis of Acne Vulgaris and the Mode of Isotretinoin Action." *G. Ital. Dermatol. Venereol.* 2010; 145(5):559–572.

Alzheimer's Disease

1. Dahm, Rolf. "Finding Alzheimer's Disease." *Am. Sci.* 2010; 98:148–155.

2. Doraiswamy, P. Murali, Gwyther, Lisa P., and Adler, Tina. *The Alzheimer's Action Plan: The Experts' Guide to the Best Diagnosis and Treatment for Memory Problems.* New York: St. Martin's Press, 2008, pp. 22–23.

3. Ishwayna, T. J., Ely, E. W., et al. "Long-term Cognitive Impairment and Functional Disability Among Survivors of Severe Sepsis." *JAMA* 2010; 304(16):1787–1794.

4. Doraiswamy, et al., op. cit., 33–34.

5. FDA Alert 6/16/08: Information for Health Professionals: Conventional Antipsychotics. http://www.fda.gov/Drugs/DrugSafety/PostmarketDrugSafetyInformationfor-PatientsandProviders/ucm124830.htm. Accessed Oct. 27, 2010.

6. Salzman, C., Jeste, D. V., et al. "Elderly Patients with Dementia-Related Symptoms of Severe Agitation and Aggression: Consensus Statement on Treatment Options, Clinical Trials Methodology, and Policy." *J. Clin. Psychiatry.* 2008; 69(6):889–898.

7. Doraiswamy, et al., op. cit., pp. 129–132.

8. Hansen, R. A., Gartlehner, G., et al. "Drug Class Review on Alzheimer's Drugs: Final Report [Internet]." Portland (OR): Oregon Health & Science University, June 2006 Drug Class Reviews.

9. AD2000 Collaborative Group. "Long-Term Donepezil Treatment in 565 Patients with Alzheimer's Disease (AD2000): Randomised Double-blind Trial." *Lancet* 2004; 363(9427):2105–2115.

10. Ibid.

11. Birks, J. "Cholinesterase Inhibitors for Alzheimer's Disease." *Cochrane Database Syst Rev.* 2006 Jan 25; (1):CD005593.

12. Birks, J., Grimley Evans, J., et al. "Rivastigmine for Alzheimer's Disease." *Cochrane Database Syst Rev.* 2009 Apr 15; (2):CD001191.

13. Sink, Kaycee M., Thomas, Joseph, III, et al. "Dual Use of Bladder Anticholinergics and Cholinesterase Inhibitors: Long-Term Functional and Cognitive Outcomes." *J. Am. Geriatr. Soc.* 2008; 56:847–853.

Arthritis

1. Papathanasiou, A. "Health Status of the Neolithic Population of Alepotrypa Cave, Greece." *Am. J. Phys. Anthropol.* 2005; 126(4):377–390.

2. Arthritis Foundation (http://www.arthritis.org), citing Helmick, C., Felson, D., et al. "Estimates of the Prevalence of Arthritis and Other Rheumatic Conditions in the United States." *Arthritis Rheum.* 2008; 58(1):15–25.

3. Berger, J. S., Brown, D. L., et al. "Aspirin Use, Dose, and Clinical Outcomes in Postmenopausal Women with Stable Cardiovascular Disease: The Women's Health Initiative Observational Study." *Circ. Cardiovasc. Qual. Outcomes.* 2009; 2(2):78–87.

4. Razzouk, L., Mathew, V., et al. "Aspirin Use Is Associated with an Improved Long-Term Survival in an Unselected Population Presenting with Unstable Angina." *Clin. Cardiol.* 2010; 33(9):553–558.

5. Wolff, T., Miller, T., and Ko, S. "Aspirin for the Primary Prevention of Cardiovascular Events: An Update of the Evidence for the U.S. Preventive Services Task Force [Internet]." Rockville, MD: Agency for Healthcare Research and Quality (US); 2009 March Report No. 09-05129-EF-1. U.S. Preventive Services Task Force Evidence Syntheses.

6. Rothwell, P. M., Wilson, M., et al. "Long-Term Effect of Aspirin on Colorectal Cancer Incidence and Mortality: 20-Year Follow-up of Five Randomised Trials." *Lancet.* 2010; 376:1741–1750.

7. Pandeya, N., Webb, P. M., et al. "Gastro-oesophageal Reflux Symptoms and the Risks of Oesophageal Cancer: Are the Effects Modified by Smoking, NSAIDs or Acid Suppressants?" *Gut.* 2010; 59(1):31–38.

8. Harris, R. E., Beebe-Donk, J., et al. "Aspirin, Ibuprofen, and Other Non-steroidal Anti-inflammatory Drugs in Cancer Prevention: A Critical Review of Non-selective COX-2 Blockade (Review)." *Oncol. Rep.* 2005; 13(4):559–583.

9. Wolfe, M. M., Lichtenstein, D. R., and Singh, G. "Gastrointestinal Toxicity of Nonsteroidal Anti-Inflammatory Drugs." *N. Engl. J. Med.* 1999; 340(24):1888–1899.

10. Topol, E. J. "Failing the Public Health: Rofecoxib, Merck, and the FDA." *N. Engl. J. Med.* 2004; 351:1707–1709.

11. Goozner, M. "What Went Wrong? FDA Veteran David Graham Speaks Out on the Drug Safety Dilemma." *AARP Bulletin,* Feb. 2005.

12. Chou, R., Helfand, M., et al. "Comparative Effectiveness and Safety of Analgesics for Osteoarthritis [Internet]." Rockville, MD: Agency for Healthcare Research and Quality (US). 2006 Sept. Report No. 06-EHC009-EF. http://www.effectivehealthcare.ahrq.gov/ehc/products/2/65/AnalgesicsFinal.pdf.

13. Baraf, H. S., Gold, M. S., et al. "Safety and Efficacy of Topical Diclofenac Sodium 1% Gel in Knee Osteoarthritis: A Randomized Controlled Trial." *Phys. Sportsmed.* 2010; 38(2):19–28.

14. Makris, U. E., Kohler, M. J., and Fraenkel, L. "Adverse Effects of Topical Nonsteroidal Antiinflammatory Drugs in Older Adults with Osteoarthritis: A Systematic Literature Review." *J. Rheumatol.* 2010; 37(6):1236–1243.

15. Coombes, B. K., Bisset, L., and Vicenzino, B. "Efficacy and Safety of Corticosteroid Injections and Other Injections for Management of Tendinopathy: A Systematic Review of Randomised Controlled Trials." *Lancet,* 2010. E-pub online ahead of print, 2010; 376:1751–1767.

16. Swindells, M. G., Logan, A. J., et al. "The Benefit of Radiologically-Guided Steroid Injections for Trapeziometacarpal Osteoarthritis." *Ann. R. Coll. Surg. Engl.* 2010; 92(8):680–684.

17. Cunnington, J., Marshall, N., et al. "A Randomized, Double-Blind, Controlled Study of Ultrasound-Guided Corticosteroid Injection into the Joint of Patients with Inflammatory Arthritis." *Arthritis Rheum.* 2010; 62(7):1862–1869.

18. Personal communication, Sept. 29, 2009, from Joanne Jordan, MD, MPH, Herman and Louise Smith Distinguished Professor of Medicine and Director of the Thurston Arthritis Research Center. Dr. Jordan is also Chief of the Division of Rheumatology, Allergy and Immunology and adjunct associate professor of epidemiology at the School of Medicine of the University of North Carolina at Chapel Hill.

19. Wandel, S., Juni, P., et al. "Effects of Glucosamine, Chondroitin, or Placebo in Patients with Osteoarthritis of Hip or Knee: Network Meta-analysis." *BMJ* 2010; 341:c4675; Doi: 10.1136/bmj.c4675. http://www.bmj.com/content/341/bmj.c4675.full.

20. Langworthy, M. J., Saad, A., and Langworthy, N. M. "Conservative Treatment Modalities and Outcomes for Osteoarthritis: The Concomitant Pyramid of Treatment." *Phys. Sportsmed.* 2010; 38(2):133–145.

21. Petrella, R. J. "Hyaluronic Acid for the Treatment of Knee Osteoarthritis: Long-Term Outcomes from a Naturalistic Primary Care Experience." *Am. J. Phys. Med. Rehabil.* 2005; 84(4):278–283.

Asthma

1. "Asthma: A Presentation of Asthma Management and Prevention." CDC. http://www.cdc.gov/asthma/speakit/default.htm. Accessed Nov. 9, 2010.

2. Hahn, D. L. "Treatment of *Chlamydia pneumoniae* Infection in Adult Asthma: A Before-After Trial." *J. Fam. Pract.* 1995; 41:345–351

3. "Epinephrine CFC Metered-Dose Inhalers—Questions and Answers." FDA. http://www.fda.gov/Drugs/DrugSafety/InformationbyDrugClass/ucm080427.htm. Accessed April 20, 2011.

4. Salpeter, S. R., Buckley, N. S., et al. "Meta-Analysis: Effect of Long-Acting Beta-Agonists on Severe Asthma Exacerbations and Asthma-Related Deaths." *Ann. Intern. Med.* 2006; 144(12):904–912.

5. Salpeter, S. R., Wall, A. J., and Buckley, N. S. "Long-Acting Beta-Agonists with and Without Inhaled Corticosteroids and Catastrophic Asthma Events." *Am. J. Med.* 2010; 123(4):322–328.

6. Cates, C. J., and Cates, M. J. "Regular Treatment with Salmeterol for Chronic Asthma: Serious Adverse Events." *Cochrane Database Syst. Rev.* 2008 Jul 15; (3):CD006363.

7. Cates, C. J., Cates, M. J., and Lasserson, T. J. "Regular Treatment with Formoterol for Chronic Asthma: Serious Adverse Events." *Cochrane Database Syst Rev.* 2008 Oct 8; (4):CD006923.

8. "Long-Acting Beta-Agonists (LABAs) Label Change." FDA. http://www.fda.gov/Safety/MedWatch/SafetyInformation/ucm218833.htm. Accessed Nov. 12, 2010.

9. Salpeter, Shelley, MD. Personal communication, April 12, 2010.

10. Salpeter, S. R. "An Update on the Safety of Long-Acting Beta-Agonists in Asthma Patients Using Inhaled Corticosteroids." *Expert Opin. Drug Saf.* 2010; 9(3):407–419.

11. Kersten, E. T., Driessen, J. M., et al. "Pilot Study: The Effect of Reducing Treatment on Exercise Induced Bronchoconstriction." *Pediatr. Pulmonol.* 2010; 45(9):927–933.

12. Singh, S., Amin, A. V., and Loke, Y. K. "Long-Term Use of Inhaled Corticosteroids and the Risk of Pneumonia in Chronic Obstructive Pulmonary Disease: A Meta-analysis." *Arch. Intern. Med.* 2009; 169(3):219–229.

13. Opat, A. J., Cohen, M. M., et al. "A Clinical Trial of the Buteyko Breathing Technique in Asthma as Taught by a Video." *J. Asthma* 2000; 37(7):557–564.

14. Cowie, R. L., Conley, D. P., et al. "A Randomised Controlled Trial of the Buteyko Technique as an Adjunct to Conventional Management of Asthma." *Respir. Med.* 2008; 102(5):726–732.

Attention Deficit Disorder (ADD)

1. Hallowell, E. M., and Ratey, J. J. *Delivered from Distraction.* New York: Random House, 2005.

2. Brimble, M. J. "Diagnosis and Management of ADHD: A New Way Forward?" *Community Pract.* 2009; 82:34–37.

3. "How to Help a Child with ADHD." *Consumer Reports,* Oct. 2010, p. 8.

4. Kemper, Kathy. Personal communication, Sept. 22, 2010.

5. Sorgi, P. J, Hallowell, E. M, et al. "Effects of an Open-Label Pilot Study with High-Dose EPA/DHA Concentrates on Plasma Phospholipids and Behavior in Children with Attention Deficit Hyperactivity Disorder." *Nutr. J.* 2007; 6:16.

6. Gevensleben, H., Holl, B., et al. "Is Neurofeedback an Efficacious Treatment for ADHD? A Randomised Controlled Clinical Trial." *J. Child. Psychol. Psychiatry.* 2009; 50(7):780–789.

7. Safren, S, A., Sprich, S., et al. "Cognitive Behavioral Therapy vs. Relaxation with Educational Support for Medication-Treated Adults with ADHD and Persistent Symptoms: A Randomized Controlled Trial." *JAMA* 2010; 304(8):875–880.

8. Bukstein, O. G., "Clinical Practice Guidelines for Attention-Deficit/Hyperactivity Disorder: A Review." *Postgrad. Med.* 2010; 122(5):69–77.

Back Pain

1. Hadler, Nortin. *Stabbed in the Back: Confronting Back Pain in an Overtreated Society.* Chapel Hill, NC: University of North Carolina Press, 2009.

2. Sarno, John, MD, attending physician at the Howard A. Rusk Institute of rehabilitation medicine at New York University Medical Center and professor of clinical rehabilitation medicine at NYU School of Medicine. Personal communication, May 17, 2010.

Breast Cancer

1. CDC "Breast Cancer Statistics." http://www.cdc.gov/cancer/breast/statistics/index.htm. Accessed Nov. 15, 2010.

2. Mandelblatt, J. S., Cronin, K. A., et al. "Effects of Mammography Screening Under Different Screening Schedules: Model Estimates of Potential Benefits and Harms." *Ann. Intern. Med.* 2009; 151(10):738–747.

3. "Implementing Comparative Effectiveness Research: Lessons from the Mammography Screening Controversy," *Science Daily* June 23, 2010. http://www.sciencedaily.com/releases/2010/06/100622165900.htm. Accessed Nov. 15, 2010.

4. Hellquist, B. N., Duffy, S. W., et al. "Effectiveness of Population-Based Service Screening with Mammography for Women Ages 40 to 49 Years: Evaluation of the Swedish Mammography Screening in Young Women (SCRY) Cohort." *Cancer* 2011; 117:714–722.

5. Susan Love, MD, president of the Dr. Susan Love Research Foundation, clinical professor of surgery at UCLA and author of *Dr. Susan Love's Breast Book*. Personal communication, Nov. 3, 2010.

6. Domchek, S. M., Friebel, T. M., et al. "Association of Risk-Reducing Surgery in BRCA1 or BRCA2 Mutation Carriers with Cancer Risk and Mortality." *JAMA* 2010; 304(9):967–975.

7. Lostumbo, L., Carbine, N. E., and Wallace, J. "Prophylactic Mastectomy for the Prevention of Breast Cancer." *Cochrane Database Syst.* Rev. 2010 Nov. 10; 11:CD002748.

Celiac Disease

1. Katz, S., and Weinerman, S. "Osteoporosis and Gastrointestinal Disease." *Gastroenterol. Hepatol. (NY)* 2010; 6(8):506–517.

2. Bürk, K., Farecki, M. L., et al. "Neurological Symptoms in Patients with Biopsy Proven Celiac Disease." *Mov. Disord.* 2009; 24(16):2358–2362.

3. Hadjivassiliou, M., Sanders, D. S., et al. "Gluten Sensitivity: From Gut to Brain." *Lancet Neurol.* 2010; 9(3):318–330.

4. Beers, M. H., Porter, R. S., et al, eds. *The Merck Manual of Diagnosis and Therapy*, 18th ed. Whitehouse Station, NJ: Merck Research Laboratories, 2006.

5. Mustalahti, K., Catassi, C., et al. "The Prevalence of Celiac Disease in Europe: Results of a Centralized, International Mass Screening Project." *Ann. Med.* 2010; 42(8):587–595.

6. Catassi, C., Kryszak, D., et al. "Natural History of Celiac Disease Autoimmunity in a USA Cohort Followed Since 1974." *Ann. Med.* 2010; 42(7):530–538.

7. Tursi, A., Elisei, W., et al. "Prevalence of Celiac Disease and Symptoms in Relatives of Patients with Celiac Disease." *Eur. Rev. Med. Pharmacol Sci.* 2010; 14(6):567–572.

8. Biagi, F., Klersy, C., et al. "Are We Not Over-estimating the Prevalence of Coeliac Disease in the General Population?" *Ann. Med.* 2010; 42(8):557–561.

9. Reeves, G. E., Squance, M. L., et al. "Diagnostic Accuracy of Coeliac Serological Tests: A Prospective Study." *Eur. J. Gastroenterol. Hepatol.* 2006; 18(5):493–501.

10. Gonzalez, S., Gupta, A., et al. "Prospective Study of the Role of Duodenal Bulb Biopsies in the Diagnosis of Celiac Disease." *Gastrointest. Endosc.* 2010; 72(4):758–765.

11. Catassi, C., and Fasano, A. "Celiac Disease Diagnosis: Simple Rules Are Better Than Complicated Algorithms." *Am. J. Med.* 2010; 123(8):691–693.

12. Campanella, J., Biagi, F., et al. "Clinical Response to Gluten Withdrawal Is Not an Indicator of Coeliac Disease." *Scand. J. Gastroenterol.* 2008; 43(11):1311–1314.

13. Chandesris, M. O., Malamut, G., et al. "Enteropathy-Associated T-Cell Lymphoma: A Review on Clinical Presentation, Diagnosis, Therapeutic Strategies and Perspectives." *Gastroenterol. Clin. Biol.* 2010; 34(11):590–605.

Deep Vein Thrombosis (DVT)

1. Tapson, V. F. "Prophylaxis Strategies for Patients with Acute Venous Thromboembolism." *Am. J. Manag. Care* 2001; 7(17 Suppl):S524-S531.

2. Philips, Jr., R. L., et al. "Learning from Malpractice Claims About Negligent, Adverse Events in Primary Care in the United States." *Qual. Saf. Health Care* 2004; 13:121–126.

3. Schiff, G. D., et al. "Diagnostic Error in Medicine." *Arch. Intern. Med.* 2009; 169:1881–1887.

4. Centers for Disease Control and Prevention. "Deep Vein Thrombosis (DVT): Health Care Professionals: Data & Statistics." http://www.cdc.gov/ncbddd/dvt/hcp _data.htm. Accessed Nov. 27, 2010.

5. Abad Rico, J. I., et al. "Overview of Venous Thromboembolism." *Drugs* 2010; 70 (Suppl.2):3–10.

6. Anderson, F. A., et al. "A Population-Perspective of the Hospital Incidence and Case Fatality Rates of Deep Vein Thrombosis and Pulmonary Embolism. The Worcester DVT Study." *Arch. Intern. Med.* 1991; 151:933–938.

7. Raskob, G. E., et al. "Surveillance for Deep Vein Thrombosis and Pulmonary Embolism: Recommendations from a National Workshop." *Am. J. Prev. Med.* 2010; 38 (4 Suppl.):S502–S509.

8. Ortel, Thomas, professor of medicine and pathology at Duke University Medical Center, medical director of the Hemostasis and Thrombosis Center at Duke, and medical director of the Clinical Coagulation Laboratory and the Platelet Antibody Laboratory at Duke, as well as the Duke Anticoagulation Clinic. He is the author (with Andra James, MD, and Victor Tapson, MD) of *100 Questions and Answers about Deep Vein Thrombosis and Pulmonary Embolism.* Personal communication, June 29, 2009.

Depression

1. Press Releases, "IMS Health Reports U.S. Prescription Sales Grew 5.1 Percent in 2009, to $300.3 Billion." April 1, 2010. http://www.imshealth.com/portal/site/ imshealth/menuitem.a46c6d4df3db4b3d88f611019418c22a/?vgnextoid=d690a27e9d5 b7210VgnVCM100000ed152ca2RCRD&cpsextcurrchannel=1.

2. Fournier, J. C., et al. "Antidepressant Drug Effects and Depression Severity." *JAMA* 2010; 303:47–53.

3. Ibid.

4. Kirsch, I., et al. "Initial Severity and Antidepressant Benefits: A Meta-Analysis of Data Submitted to the Food and Drug Administration." *PLoS Med.* 2008; 5:e45.

5. Begley, Sharon. "The Depressing News About Antidepressants." *Newsweek,* Jan. 29, 2010.

6. Personal communication from Stephen Ilardi, associate professor of clinical psychology at the University of Kansas, May 29, 2010. His book is *The Depression Cure: The 6-Step Program to Beat Depression Without Drugs.*

7. Ibid.

Diabetes

1. American Diabetes Association Diabetes Basics, "Diabetes Statistics." http:// www.diabetes.org/diabetes-basics/diabetes-statistics. Accessed Nov. 25, 2010.

2. Centers for Disease Control and Prevention, "Older, More Diverse Population and Longer Lifespans Contribute to Increase." Press release, Oct. 22, 2010. http://www.cdc.gov/media/pressrel/2010/r101022.html. Accessed Nov. 25, 2010.

3. American Heart Association, "What Is the Metabolic Syndrome?" http://www.americanheart.org/presenter.jhtml?identifier=4756. Accessed, Nov. 25, 2010.

4. UnitedHealth Group, "The United States of Diabetes: Challenges and Opportunities in the Decade Ahead." Working Paper 5, Nov. 2010. http://www.unitedhealthgroup.com/hrm/UNH_WorkingPaper5.pdf. Accessed Nov. 25, 2010.

5. Patel, C. J., et al. "An Environment-Wide Association Study (EWAS) on Type 2 Diabetes Mellitus." *PLoS One,* 2010; 5:e10746.

6. Chang, J. W., et al. "Simultaneous Exposure of Non-Diabetics to High Levels of Dioxins and Mercury Increases Their Risk of Insulin Resistance." *J. Hazard. Mater.* 2011; 185:749–755.

7. Alonso-Magdalena, P., et al. "Bisphenol-A: A New Diabetogenic Factor?" *Hormones* (Athens) 2010; 9:118–126.

8. Ropero, A. B., et al. "Bisphenol-A Disruption of the Endocrine Pancreas and Blood Glucose Homeostasis." *Int. J. Androl.* 2008; 31:194–200.

9. Alonso-Magdalena, P., et al. "Bisphenol-A Exposure During Pregnancy Disrupts Glucose Homeostasis in Mothers and Adult Male Offspring." *Environ. Health Perspect.* 2010; 118:1243–1250.

10. Stahlhut, R. W., et al. "Concentrations of Urinary Phthalate Metabolites Are Associated with Increased Waist Circumference and Insulin Resistance in Adult U.S. Males." *Environ. Health Perspect.* 2007; 115:876–882.

11. Samuel, V. T. "Fructose Induced Lipogenesis: From Sugar to Fat to Insulin Resistance." *Trends Endocrinol. Metabol.* 2011; 22:60–65.

12. Bray, G. A. "Fructose: Pure, White, and Deadly? Fructose, by Any Other Name, Is a Health Hazard." *J. Diabetes Sci. Technol.* 2010; 4:1003–1007.

13. Stanhole, K. L., and Havel, P. J. "Endocrine and Metabolic Effects of Consuming Beverages Sweetened with Fructose, Glucose, Sucrose, or High-Fructose Corn Syrup." *Am. J. Clin. Nutr.* 2008; 88:1733S–1737S.

14. Sluijs, I., et al. "Carbohydrate Quantity and Quality and Risk of Type 2 Diabetes in the European Prospective Investigation Into Cancer and Nutrition—Netherlands (EPIC-NL) Study." *Am. J. Clin. Nutr.* 2010; 92:905–911.

15. Barclay, A. W., et al. "Glycemic Index, Glycemic Load, and Chronic Disease Risk—A Meta-Analysis of Observational Studies." *Am. J. Clin. Nutr.* 2008; 87:627–637.

16. Bernstein, R. K. *Dr. Bernstein's Diabetes Solution, Revised and Updated: The Complete Guide to Achieving Normal Blood Sugars.* Boston: Little, Brown, 2003.

17. Brand-Miller, J., Wolever, T. M. S., et al. *The New Glucose Revolution: The Authoritative Guide to the Glycemic Index—The Dietary Solution for Lifelong Health.* New York: Marlowe, 2003.

18. Brand-Miller, J., Wolever, T. M. S., et al. *The Low GI Handbook: The New Glucose Revolution Guide to the Long-Term Health Benefits of Low GI Eating.* Philadelphia, PA: Da Capo Press, 2010.

19. ACCORD Study Group, "Effects of Combination Lipid Therapy in Type 2 Diabetes Mellitus." *N. Engl. J. Med.* 2010; 362:1563–1574.

20. ACCORD Study Group, "Effects of Intensive Blood-Pressure Control in Type 2 Diabetes." *N. Engl. J. Med.* 2010; 362:1575–1585.

21. Cooper-DeHoff, R. M., et al. "Tight Blood Pressure Control and Cardiovascular Outcomes Among Hypertensive Patients with Diabetes and Coronary Artery Disease." *JAMA* 2010; 304:61–68.

22. The Action to Control Cardiovascular Risk in Diabetes Study Group. "Effects of Intensive Glucose Lowering in Type 2 Diabetes." *N. Engl. J. Med.* 2008; 358:2545–2559.

23. Nilsson, P. M. "ACCORD and Risk-Factor Control in Type 2 Diabetes." *N. Engl. J. Med.* 2010; 362:1628–1630.

24. Currie, C. J., et al. "Survival as a Function of HbA1c in People with Type 2 Diabetes: A Retrospective Cohort Study." *Lancet* 2010; 375:481–495.

25. Harris, G. "Caustic Government Report Deals Blow to Diabetes Drug." *New York Times,* July 9, 2010.

26. Nissen, S. E., and Wolski, K. "Rosiglitazone Revisited: An Updated Meta-Analysis of Risk for Myocardial Infarction and Cardiovascular Mortality." *Arch. Int. Med.* 2010; 303:1196–1198.

27. Goldner, M. G., et al. "Effects of Hypoglycemic Agents on Vascular Complications in Patients with Adult-Onset Diabetes: III. Clinical Implications of the UGDP Results." *JAMA* 1971; 218:1400–1410.

28. Gilbert, J. P., et al. "Report of the Committee for the Assessment of Biometric Aspects of Controlled Trials of Hypoglycemic Agents." *JAMA* 1975; 231:583–608.

Fibromyalgia

1. Chakrabarty, S., and Zoorob, R. "Fibromyalgia." *Am. Fam. Physician.* 2007; 76(2):247–254.

2. National Fibromyalgia Association. http://www.fmaware.org. Accessed Nov. 26, 2010.

3. Mease, P. "Fibromyalgia Syndrome: Review of Clinical Presentation, Pathogenesis, Outcome Measures, and Treatment." *J. Rheumatol. Suppl.* 2005; 75:6–21.

4. Teitelbaum, Jacob, MD, medical director of the Fibromyalgia and Fatigue Centers. Personal communication, Feb. 27, 2009.

5. Di Franco, M., Iannuccelli, C., and Valesini, G. "Neuroendocrine Immunology of Fibromyalgia." *Ann. NY Acad. Sci.* 2010; 1193:84–90.

6. Ablin, J. N., and Buskila, D. "Emerging Therapies for Fibromyalgia: An Update." *Expert Opin. Emerg. Drugs.* 2010: 15(3):521–533.

7. Kyle, J. A., Dugan, B. D., and Testerman, K. K. "Milnacipran for Treatment of Fibromyalgia." *Ann. Pharmacother.* 2010; 44(9):1422–1429.

8. Häuser, W., Petzke, F., et al. "Comparative Efficacy and Acceptability of Amitriptyline, Duloxetine and Milnacipran in Fibromyalgia Syndrome: A Systematic Review with Meta-analysis." *Rheumatology* (Oxford). 2011; 50:532–543.

9. Hsu, E. S. "Acute and Chronic Pain Management in Fibromyalgia: Updates on Pharmacotherapy." *Am. J. Ther.* 2010. E-pub ahead of print, May 7, 2010. http://journals .lww.com/americantherapeutics/Abstract/publishahead/Acute_and_Chronic_Pain _Management_in_Fibromyalgia_.99764.aspx.

10. Arnold, L. M., and Clauw, D. J. "Fibromyalgia Syndrome: Practical Strategies for Improving Diagnosis and Patient Outcomes." *Am. J. Med.* 2010; 123(6):S2.

11. Spaeth, M., and Briley, M. "Fibromyalgia: A Complex Syndrome Requiring a Multidisciplinary Approach." *Hum. Psychopharmacol.* 2009; 24 Suppl 1:S3–S10.

12. Imamura, M., Cassius, D. A., and Fregni, F. "Fibromyalgia: From Treatment to Rehabilitation." *Eur. J. Pain.* 2009; 3(2):117–122.

13. Sarzi-Puttini, P., Atzeni, F., and Cazzola, M. "Neuroendocrine Therapy of Fibro-myalgia Syndrome: An Update." *Ann. NY Acad. Sci.* 2010; 1193:91–97.

14. Wang, C., Schmid, C. H., et al. "A Randomized Trial of Tai Chi for Fibromyal-gia." *N. Engl. J. Med.* 2010; 363(8):743–754.

15. Carson, J. W., Carson, K. M., et al. "A Pilot Randomized Controlled Trial of the Yoga of Awareness Program in the Management of Fibromyalgia." *Pain* 2010; 151(2):530–539.

16. Busch, A. J., Barber, K. A., et al. "Exercise for Treating Fibromyalgia Syndrome." *Cochrane Database Syst. Rev.* 2007 Oct 17; (4):CD003786.

17. Teitelbaum, J. E., Johnson, C., and St. Cyr, J. "The Use of D-Ribose in Chronic Fatigue Syndrome and Fibromyalgia: A Pilot Study." *J. Altern. Complement. Med.* 2006; 12(9):857–862.

18. De Silva, V., El-Metwally, A., et al. "Evidence for the Efficacy of Complementary and Alternative Medicines in the Management of Fibromyalgia: A Systematic Review." *Rheumatology* (Oxford). 2010; 49(6):1063–1068.

Heartburn

1. Nicholas Shaheen, MD, MPH, professor of medicine and epidemiology at the UNC School of Medicine and UNC School of Public Health, and director of the UNC Center for Esophageal Diseases and Swallowing. Personal communication, Jan. 14, 2010.

2. Shaheen, N. J., Madanick, R. D., et al. "Gastroesophageal Reflux Disease as an Etiology of Sleep Disturbance in Subjects with Insomnia and Minimal Reflux Symp-toms: A Pilot Study of Prevalence and Response to Therapy." *Dig. Dis. Sci.* 2008; 53(6):1493–1499.

3. Moazzez, R., Bartlett, D., and Anggiansah, A. "The Effect of Chewing Sugar-Free Gum on Gastro-Esophageal Reflux." *J. Dent. Res.* 2005; 84(11):1062–1065.

4. Austin, G. L., Thiny, M. T., et al. "A Very Low-Carbohydrate Diet Improves Gas-troesophageal Reflux and its Symptoms." *Dig. Dis. Sci.* 2006; 51(8):1307–1312.

5. Ali, T., Roberts, D. N., and Tierney, W. M. "Long-Term Safety Concerns with Proton Pump Inhibitors." *Am. J. Med.* 2009; 122(10):896–903.

6. Yang, Y. X., Lewis, J. D., et al. "Long-term Proton Pump Inhibitor Therapy and Risk of Hip Fracture." *JAMA* 2006; 296(24):2947–2953.

7. Targownik, L. E., Lix, L. M., et al. "Use of Proton Pump Inhibitors and Risk of Osteoporosis-Related Fractures." *CMAJ* 2008; 179(4):319–326.

8. Laheij, R. J., Sturkenboom, M. C., et al. "Risk of Community-Acquired Pneumonia and Use of Gastric Acid-Suppressive Drugs." *JAMA* 2004; 292(16):1955–1960.

9. Canani, R. B., Cirillo, P., et al. "Therapy with Gastric Acidity Inhibitors Increases the Risk of Acute Gastroenteritis and Community-Acquired Pneumonia in Children." *Pediatrics* 2006; 117(5):c817-e820.

10. Dublin, S., Walker, R. L., et al. "Use of Proton Pump Inhibitors and H2 Blockers and Risk of Pneumonia in Older Adults: A Population-Based Case-Control Study." *Pharmacoepidemiol. Drug Saf.* 2010; 19(8):792–802.

11. Howell, M. D., Novack, V., et al. "Iatrogenic Gastric Acid Suppression and the Risk of Nosocomial *Clostridium difficile* Infection." *Arch. Intern. Med.* 2010; 170(9):784–790.

12. Heidelbaugh, J. J., Goldberg, K. L., and Inadomi, J. M. "Overutilization of Proton Pump Inhibitors: A Review of Cost-effectiveness and Risk [Corrected]." *Am. J. Gastroenterol.* 2009; 104 Suppl 2:S27-S32.

13. Reimer, C., Søndergaard, B., et al. "Proton-Pump Inhibitor Therapy Induces Acid-Related Symptoms in Healthy Volunteers after Withdrawal of Therapy." *Gastroenterology* 2009; 137(1):80–87.

14. Kwok, C. S., Nijjar, R. S., and Loke, Y. K. "Effects of Proton Pump Inhibitors on Adverse Gastrointestinal Events in Patients Receiving Clopidogrel: Systematic Review and Meta-analysis." *Drug Saf.* 2011; 34:47–57.

15. Oyetayo, O. O., and Talbert, R. L. "Proton Pump Inhibitors and Clopidogrel: Is It a Significant Drug Interaction?" *Expert Opin. Drug Saf.* 2010; 9(4):593–602.

16. Laine, L., and Hennekens, C. "Proton Pump Inhibitor and Clopidogrel Interaction: Fact or Fiction?" *Am. J. Gastroenterol.* 2010; 105(1):34–41.

17. Charlot, M., Ahlehoff, O., et al. "Proton-Pump Inhibitors Are Associated with Increased Cardiovascular Risk Independent of Clopidogrel Use: A Nationwide Cohort Study." *Ann. Intern. Med.* 2010; 153(6):378–386.

Hypothyroidism

1. Norman, J. "Hypothyroidism: Too Little Thyroid Hormone." *Endocrine Web* 3/29/2009–4/19/2011. http://www.endocrineweb.com/conditions/thyroid/hypo thyroidism-too-little-thyroid-hormone. Accessed Nov. 27, 2010.

2. Shomon, M. *Living Well with Hypothyroidism: What Your Doctor Doesn't Tell You . . . That You Need to Know.* New York: HarperResource, 2005.

3. Shomon, Mary. Personal communication, Aug. 1, 2009.

4. Shomon, M. "Thyroid Testing: What Is a Normal TSH Level?" About.com, Feb. 25, 2010. http://thyroid.about.com/od/gettestedanddiagnosed/a/normaltshlevel.htm. Accessed Nov. 27, 2010.

5. Razvi, S., et al. "Subclinical Thyroid Disorders: Significance and Clinical Impact." *J. Clin. Pathol.* 2010; 63:379–386.

6. Lohr, A. "To Treat or Not to Treat: New Data Says a Mild Case of Underactive Thyroid Disease Should Be Left Alone." Endocrine Society, June 16, 2008. http://www.endo-society.org/media/press/2006/jan06thyroid.cfm. Accessed Nov. 27, 2010.

7. Waise, A., and Price, H. C. "The Upper Limit of the Reference Range for Thyroid-Stimulating Hormone Should Not Be Confused with a Cut-off to Define Subclinical Hypothyroidism." *Ann. Clin. Biochem.* 2009; 46(Pt 2):93–98.

8. Jones, D. D., May, K. E., and Geraci, S. A. "Subclinical Thyroid Disease." *Am. J. Med.* 2010; 123(6):502–504.

9. Rodondi, N., den Elzen, W. P., et al. "Subclinical Hypothyroidism and the Risk of Coronary Heart Disease and Mortality." *JAMA* 2010; 304(12):1365–1374.

10. Parle, J., Roberts, L., et al. "A Randomized Controlled Trial of the Effect of Thyroxine Replacement on Cognitive Function in Community-Living Elderly Subjects with Subclinical Hypothyroidism: The Birmingham Elderly Thyroid Study." *J. Clin. Endocrinol. Metab.* 2010; 95(8):3623–3632.

11. Bunevicius, R., Kazanavicius, G., et al. "Effects of Thyroxine as Compared with Thyroxine Plus Triiodothyronine in Patients with Hypothyroidism." *N. Engl. J. Med.* 1999; 340(6):424–429.

12. Clyde, P. W., Harari, A. E., et al. "Combined Levothyroxine Plus Liothyronine Compared with Levothyroxine Alone in Primary Hypothyroidism: A Randomized Controlled Trial." *JAMA* 2003; 290(22):2952–2958.

13. Siegmund, W., Spieker, K., et al. "Replacement Therapy with Levothyroxine Plus Triiodothyronine (Bioavailable Molar Ratio 14:1) Is Not Superior to Thyroxine Alone to Improve Well-Being and Cognitive Performance in Hypothyroidism." *Clin. Endocrinol.* (Oxford) 2004; 60(6):750–757.

14. Escobar-Morreale, H. F., Botella-Carretero, J. I., et al. "Thyroid Hormone Replacement Therapy in Primary Hypothyroidism: A Randomized Trial Comparing L-Thyroxine Plus Liothyronine with L-Thyroxine Alone." *Ann. Intern. Med.* 2005; 142(6):412–424.

15. Danzi, S., and Klein, I. "Potential Uses of T3 in the Treatment of Human Disease." *Clin. Cornerstone* 2005; 7 Suppl 2:S9-S15.

16. Appelhof, B. C., Fliers, E., et al. "Combined Therapy with Levothyroxine and Liothyronine in Two Ratios, Compared with Levothyroxine Monotherapy in Primary Hypothyroidism: A Double-Blind, Randomized, Controlled Clinical Trial." *J. Clin. Endocrinol. Metab.* 2005; 90(5):2666–2674.

17. Acosta, B. M., and Bianco, A. C. "New Insights into Thyroid Hormone Replacement Therapy." *F1000 Med. Rep.* 2010 May 11; 2. pii:34.

18. Liwanpo, L., and Hershman, J. M. "Conditions and Drugs Interfering with Thyroxine Absorption." *Best Pract. Res. Clin. Endocrinol. Metab.* 2009; 23(6):781–792.

19. Ibid.

20. Bailey, D. G. "Fruit Juice Inhibition of Uptake Transport: A New Type of Food-Drug Interaction." *Br. J. Clin. Pharmacol.* 2010; 70(5):645–655.

21. Bolk, N., Visser, T. J., et al. "Effects of Evening vs Morning Thyroxine Ingestion

on Serum Thyroid Hormone Profiles in Hypothyroid Patients." *Clin. Endocrinol.* (Oxford) 2007; 66(1):43–48.

22. Shomon, op. cit., pp. 113–114.

Migraine Headache

1. Joel Saper, MD, FACP, FAAN, founder and director of the Michigan Head-Pain and Neurological Institute and professor of medicine (neurology) at Michigan State University. Personal communication, April 5, 2008.

2. Tepper, S. J., and Tepper, D. E. "Breaking the Cycle of Medication Overuse Headache." *Cleve. Clin. J. Med.* 2010; 77(4):236–242.

3. Fritsche, G., Frettloh, J., et al. "Prevention of Medication Overuse in Patients with Migraine." *Pain* 2010; 151(2):404–413.

4. Smitherman, T. A., Walters, A. B., et al. "The Use of Antidepressants for Headache Prophylaxis." *CNS Neurosci. Ther.* 2010. E-pub ahead of print, July 2010. http://onlinelibrary.wiley.com/doi/10.1111/j.1755-5949.2010.00170.x/abstract.

5. Diener, H. C., Holle, D., and Dodick, D. "Treatment of Chronic Migraine." *Curr. Pain Headache Rep.* 2011; 15:64–69.

6. Saper, op. cit.

7. Barra, S., Lanero, S., et al. "Sumatriptan Therapy for Headache and Acute Myocardial Infarction." *Expert Opin. Pharmacother.* 2010; 11(16):2727–2737.

Osteoporosis

1. NIH Osteoporosis and Related Bone Diseases National Resource Center: Osteoporosis Overview. http://www.niams.nih.gov/Health_Info/Bone/Osteoporosis/overview.asp. Accessed Nov. 6, 2010.

2. Lapcevic, W. A., French, D. D., and Campbell, R. R. "All-Cause Mortality Rates of Hip Fractures Treated in the VHA: Do They Differ from Medicare Facilities?" *J. Am. Med. Dir. Assoc.* 2010; 11(2):116–119.

3. Young, Y., Fried, L. P., and Kuo, Y. H. "Hip Fractures Among Elderly Women: Longitudinal Comparison of Physiological Function Changes and Health Care Utilization. " *J. Am. Med. Dir. Assoc.* 2010; 11(2):100–105.

4. Moynihan, R., and Cassels, A. *Selling Sickness: How the World's Biggest Pharmaceutical Companies Are Turning Us All into Patients.* New York: Nation Books, 2005.

5. Lindner, B. "Long-Term Fosamax Use May Cause Brittle Bones in Some Women. Mar. 10, 2010. Digital Journal. http://www.digitaljournal.com/article/288892. Accessed Nov. 6, 2010.

6. Sato, Y., Iwamoto, J., and Honda, Y. "Amelioration of Osteoporosis and Hypovitaminosis D by Sunlight Exposure in Parkinson's Disease." *Parkinsonism Relat. Disord.* 2011; 17:22–26.

7. Lips, P., Bouillon, R., et al. "Reducing Fracture Risk with Calcium and Vitamin D." *Clin. Endocrinol.* (Oxford). 2010; 73(3):277–285.

8. Bolland, M. J., Avenell, A., et al. "Effect of Calcium Supplements on Risk of Myocardial Infarction and Cardiovascular Events: Meta-analysis." *BMJ* 2010; 341:c3691.

9. Allen, M. R., and Burr, D. B. "Bisphosphonate Effects on Bone Turnover, Microdamage, and Mechanical Properties: What We Think We Know and What We Know That We Don't Know." *Bone* 2010. E-pub ahead of print, Oct. 16, 2010. www.ncbi.nlm.nih.giv/pubmed/20955825.

10. Lewiecki, E. M. "Clinical Use of Denosumab for the Treatment for Postmenopausal Osteoporosis." *Curr. Med. Res. Opin.* 2010; 26:2807–2812.

11. Mazziotti, G., Canalis, E., and Giustina, A. "Drug-Induced Osteoporosis: Mechanisms and Clinical Implications." *Am. J. Med.* 2010; 123(10):877–884.

Prostate Problems

1. Izard, J., and Nickel, J. C. "Impact of Medical Therapy on Transurethral Resection of the Prostate: Two Decades of Change." *BJU Int.* 2010. E-pub ahead of print; doi: 10.1111/j.1464–410X.2010.09737.x.

2. Smith, A. B., and Carson, C. C. "Finasteride in the Treatment of Patients with Benign Prostatic Hyperplasia: A Review." *Ther. Clin. Risk Manag.* 2009; 5(3):535–545.

3. Roehrborn, C. G., Siami, P., et al. "The Effects of Combination Therapy with Dutasteride and Tamsulosin on Clinical Outcomes in Men with Symptomatic Benign Prostatic Hyperplasia: 4-Year Results from the CombAT Study." *Eur. Urol.* 2010; 57(1):123–131.

4. Logan, Y. T., and Belgeri, M. T. "Monotherapy Versus Combination Drug Therapy for the Treatment of Benign Prostatic Hyperplasia." *Am. J. Geriatr. Pharmacother.* 2005; 3(2):103–114.

5. Al-Hussaini, Z. K., and McVary, K. T. "Alpha-Blockers and Intraoperative Floppy Iris Syndrome: Ophthalmic Adverse Events Following Cataract Surgery." *Curr. Urol. Rep.* 2010; 11(4):242–248.

6. Wilt, T. J., Macdonald, R., et al. "5-α-Reductase Inhibitors for Prostate Cancer Chemoprevention: An Updated Cochrane Systematic Review." *BJU Int.* 2010; 106(10):1444–1451.

7. Andriole, G. L., Bostwick, D. G., et al. "Effect of Dutasteride on the Risk of Prostate Cancer." *N. Engl. J. Med.* 2010; 362(13):1192–1202.

8. Wilt, T. J., MacDonald, R., et al. "Five-alpha-reductase Inhibitors for Prostate Cancer Prevention." *Cochrane Database Syst. Rev.* 2008 April 16; (2):CD007091.

9. Wilt, T., Ishani, A., and MacDonald, R. "*Serenoa repens* for Benign Prostatic Hyperplasia." *Cochrane Database Syst. Rev.* 2002; (3):CD001423.

10. Wilt, T., Ishani, A., et al. "*Pygeum africanum* for Benign Prostatic Hyperplasia." *Cochrane Database Syst. Rev.* 2002; (1):CD001044.

11. Dall'Era, M. A., Konety, B. R., et al. "Active Surveillance for the Management of Prostate Cancer in a Contemporary Cohort." *Cancer* 2008; 112(12):2664–2670.

12. Hayes, J. H., Ollendorf, D. A., et al. "Active Surveillance Compared with Initial Treatment for Men with Low-Risk Prostate Cancer." *JAMA* 2010; 304(21):2373–2380.

Tick-Borne Diseases

1. Elston, D. M. "Tick Bites and Skin Rashes." *Curr. Opin. Infect. Dis.* 2010; 23(2):132–138.

2. Breitschwerdt, Edward, DVM, professor of medicine at North Carolina State University College of Veterinary Medicine. Personal communication, March 4, 2009.

3. Woldehiwet, Z. "The Natural History of Anaplasma phagocytophilum." *Vet. Parasitol.* 2010; 167(2–4):108–122.

4. Ismail, N., Bloch, K. C., and McBride, J. W. "Human Ehrlichiosis and Anaplasmosis." *Clin. Lab. Med.* 2010; 30(1):261–292.

5. Breitschwerdt, E. B., Maggi, R. G., et al. "Bartonellosis: An Emerging Infectious Disease of Zoonotic Importance to Animals and Human Beings." *J. Vet. Emerg. Crit. Care* (San Antonio). 2010; 20(1):8–30.

Appendix 1: Top 10 List of Potentially Problematic Pills

1. Levinson, Daniel R. *Adverse Events in Hospitals: National Incidence Among Medicare Beneficiaries.* Health and Human Services, Office of Inspector General, Nov. 2010; OEI-06-09-00090.

2. Wilcox, C. M., et al. "Patterns of Use and Public Perception of Over-the-Counter Pain Relievers: Focus on Nonsteroidal Antiinflammatory Drugs." *J. Rheumatol.* 2005; 32:2218–2224.

3. Wolfe, M. M., et al. "Gastrointestinal Toxicity of Nonsteroidal Anti-Inflammatory Drugs." *N. Engl. J. Med.* 1999; 340:1888–1899.

4. U.S. Food and Drug Administration, "Margaret A. Humburg, M.D., Commissioner of Food and Drugs—Remarks at the Consumer Healthcare Products Association Annual Executive Conference." March, 20, 1020. http://www.fda.gov/NewsEvents/Speeches/ucm210009.htm. Accessed Nov. 21, 2010.

5. Forman, J. P., et al. "Frequency of Analgesic Use and Risk of Hypertension Among Men." *Arch. Intern. Med.* 2007; 167:394–399.

6. Sudano, I., et al. "Acetaminophen Increases Blood Pressure in Patients with Coronary Artery Disease." *Circulation* 2010; 122:1789–1796.

7. Launianen, T., et al. "Adverse Interaction of Warfarin and Paracetamol: Evidence from a Post-Mortem Study." *Eur. J. Clin. Pharmacol.* 2010; 66:97–103.

8. Parra, D., et al. "The Effect of Acetaminophen on the International Normalized Ratio in Patients Stabilized on Warfarin Therapy." *Pharmacotherapy* 2007; 27:675–683.

9. Sinatra, R. "Causes and Consequences of Inadequate Management of Acute Pain." *Pain Med.* 2010; 11:1859–1871.

10. Davies, E. C., et al. "Adverse Drug Reactions in Hospital In-Patients: A Prospective Analysis of 3695 Patient-Episodes." *PLoS One* 2009; 4:e4439.

11. Kane-Gill, S. L., et al. "Adverse Drug Reactions in Hospital and Ambulatory Care Settings Identified Using a Large Administrative Database." *Ann. Pharmacother.* 2010; 44:983–993.

12. The Cardiac Arrhythmia Suppression Trial CAST Investigators. "Preliminary Report of Encainide and Flecainide on Mortality in a Randomized Trial of Arrhythmia Suppression After Myocardial Infarction." *N. Engl. J. Med.* 1989; 321:406–412.

13. Lieberman, J. A., et al. "Effectiveness of Antipsychotic Drugs in Patients with Chronic Schizophrenia." *N. Engl. J. Med.* 2005; 353:1209–1223.

14. Ray, W. A., et al. "Atypical Antipsychotic Drugs and the Risk of Sudden Cardiac Death." *N. Engl. J. Med.* 2009; 360:225–235.

15. Schneider, L. S., et al. "Risk of Death with Atypical Antipsychotic Drug Treatment for Dementia." *JAMA* 2005; 292:1934–1943.

16. Gatyas, G. "IMS Health Reports U.S. Prescription Sales Grew 5.1 Percent in 2009, to $300.3 Billion." www.imshealth.com IMS Health, April 2010.

17. Vedantam, S. "Against Depression, A Sugar Pill Is Hard to Beat." *Washington Post*, May 7, 2002.

18. Khan, A., and Schwarta, K. "Study Designs and Outcomes in Antidepressant Clinical Trials." *Essent. Psychopharmacol.* 2005; 6:221–226.

19. Moncrieff, J., and Kirsch, I. "Efficacy of Antidepressants in Adults." *BMJ* 2005; 331:155–159.

20. Kirsch, I., et al. "Initial Severity and Antidepressant Benefits: A Meta-Analysis of Data Submitted to the Food and Drug Administration." *PLoS Med.* 2008; 5:e45.

Index

Joe Graedon, MS

Joe Graedon received a Bachelor of Science degree from Pennsylvania State University in 1967 and then did research on mental illness, sleep, and basic brain physiology at the New Jersey Neuropsychiatric Institute in Princeton. In 1971, he earned a Master of Science degree in pharmacology from the University of Michigan. In 2006, Joe was awarded the honorary degree of Doctor of Humane Letters from Long Island University in recognition of his work as one of the country's leading drug experts for the consumer.

Joe has lectured at the Duke University School of Nursing and the University of California, San Francisco (UCSF) School of Pharmacy. From 1971 to 1974, he taught pharmacology at the School of Medicine of the Universidad Autonoma "Benito Juárez" of Oaxaca, Mexico. He served as a consultant to the Federal Trade Commission on over-the-counter drug issues from 1978 to 1983 and was on the Advisory Board for the Drug Studies Unit at UCSF from 1983 to 1989.

Joe has been an adjunct assistant professor, Division of Pharmacy Practice and Experiential Education, at the University of North Carolina (UNC) Eshelman School of Pharmacy at Chapel Hill since 1986 and was a member of the National Policy Advisory Board for the UNC Center for Education and Research on Therapeutics (CERTS). He is a member of the American Association for the Advancement of Science (AAAS), the Society for Neuroscience, and the New York Academy of Science. In 2005, he was elected to the rank of AAAS Fellow for "exceptional contribution to the communication of the rational use of pharmaceutical products and an understanding of health issues to the public."

Joe has served as an editorial adviser to *Men's Health Newsletter* and to *Prevention* magazine. He is an advisory board member of the American Botanical Council and has served as a member of the Board of Visitors, UNC Eshelman School of Pharmacy, since 1989. He served on the Patient Safety and Clinical Quality Committee of the Duke University Health System (DUHS) Board of Directors from 2003 to 2011.

Joe's features on health and pharmaceuticals have been syndicated nationally to public television stations via the Intraregional Program Service member exchange. Joe is considered one of the country's leading drug experts for consumers and speaks frequently on issues of pharmaceuticals, nutrition, herbs, home remedies, and self-care. He has appeared as a guest on many major U.S. national television shows, including *Dateline, 20/20, The Geraldo Rivera Show, The Oprah Winfrey Show, Live with Regis and Kathie Lee, Today, Good Morning America, CBS Morning News, NBC Nightly News with Tom Brokaw, Extra, The Phil Donahue Show*, and *The Tonight Show with Johnny Carson*. A TV pledge special was underwritten by PBS in 1998. He has also coauthored a novel, *No Deadly Drug* (Pocket Books, 1992), with Tom Ferguson, MD.

Teresa Graedon, PhD

Medical anthropologist Teresa Graedon is a best-selling author, syndicated newspaper columnist, and award-winning internationally syndicated radio talk-show host. Teresa graduated magna cum laude with a Bachelor of Arts degree from Bryn Mawr College in 1969, majoring in anthropology. She attended graduate school at the University of Michigan, receiving her Master of Arts degree in 1971. She received a fellowship from the Institute for Environmental Quality (1972–1975), which enabled her to pursue doctoral research on health and nutritional status in a migrant community in Oaxaca, Mexico. Her doctorate was awarded in 1976.

Teresa taught at the Duke University School of Nursing with an adjunct appointment in the Department of Anthropology from 1975 to 1979. Thereafter she periodically taught courses in medical anthropology and international health at Duke University. From 1982 to 1983, she pursued postdoctoral training in medical anthropology at the University of California, San Francisco. With Kit Gruelle, she coauthored a cookbook, *Chocolate Without Guilt* (Graedon Enterprises, 2002).

Teresa is a fellow of the Society for Applied Anthropology, and a member of the American Anthropological Association and the Society for Medical Anthropology. She previously served on the Foundation Board of the University of North Carolina School of Nursing and the Patient Safety and Clinical Quality Committee of the Duke University Health System Board of Directors and as an editorial adviser to *Prevention* magazine.

JOE AND TERRY

For over a decade, Joe and Terry contributed a regular column on self-medication to *Medical Self-Care*, Tom Ferguson, MD's magazine. Their thrice-weekly newspaper column, *The People's Pharmacy*, has been syndicated nationally by King Features Syndicate since 1978. *The People's Pharmacy* radio show won a Silver Award from the Corporation for Public Broadcasting in 1992. It is syndicated to more than a hundred radio stations in the United States through public radio. In 2003, Joe and Teresa received the Alvarez Award at the sixty-third annual conference of the American Medical Writers Association for "Excellence in Medical Communications." Joe and Terry were named "Hometown Heroes" through Chapel Hill's WCHL Village Pride Award in 2009.

Joe and Terry were charter members of the North Carolina Consortium of Natural Medicine and Public Health and served on the Consortium Executive Committee in 2003. Joe and Terry served on the Patient Advocacy Council of Duke University Health System from 2005 to 2011, which Terry co-chaired from 2008 to 2009.

Terry and Joe were presented with the America Talks Health "Health Headliner of 1998" award for "superior contribution to the advancement of medicine and public health education." Together they have been designated Ambassadors Plenipotentiary by the City of Medicine, Durham, North Carolina, where they live. You can communicate with the Graedons through their website, www.peoplespharmacy.com.

Visit the authors at topscrewups.com.